10-Minute
Home Workouts for
Seniors

*7 Simple No Equipment Workouts for
Each Day of the Week.
70+ Illustrated Exercises with Video
Demos for Cardio, Core, Yoga, Back
Stretching, and more.*

By Brian Hardy

Not all exercises are suitable for everyone, and this or any other exercise program may result in injury. Please always consult your doctor before beginning this or any other exercise program, especially if you have any chronic or recurring condition, and/or if you are pregnant, nursing, or elderly. This exercise program is not recommended if you experience chest pains or have uncontrolled blood pressure or other uncontrolled chronic diseases. By performing any of the exercises in this program, you assume all risks of injury from doing so. The authors are not responsible or liable for any injury or loss you may sustain by participating in this exercise program. Always warm up before beginning any workout and never exercise beyond the level at which you feel comfortable. Please stop exercising immediately if you experience pain, soreness, fatigue, shortness of breath, dizziness, light-headedness, blurred vision, headache, nausea, sickness, illness, dehydration, excessive sweating, or any other discomfort. If any of these symptoms persist after you stop exercising, please seek medical help immediately. This book is made for entertainment purposes only and has no medicinal or therapeutic claims, such as claims to treat, cure, heal, or reverse a disease, addiction, or ailment. This exercise program and instructions provided in this program are not intended, and should not be used, as a substitute for professional medical advice, diagnosis or treatment. The authors makes no representation or warranty, whether express or implied, with respect to the safety, usefulness, or the result of this exercise program.

SPECIAL BONUS

Want a Workout Tracker Logbook (with Inspiring Quotes) + The Audio Guide (once released) for Free?

Updated Workout Logbook

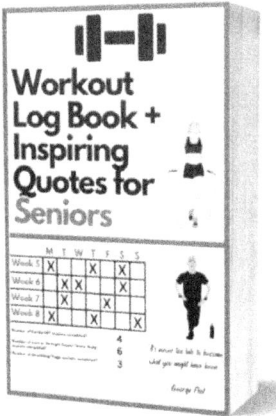

Audiobook Guide

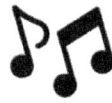

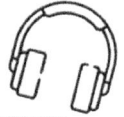

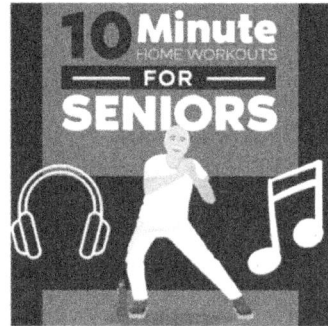

Get FREE, unlimited access to these and all of my new books by joining the community!

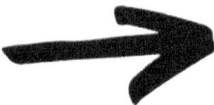

SCAN WITH YOUR PHONE CAMERA

TABLE OF CONTENTS

LEVEL 2

BRIAN HARDY

INTRODUCTION

Welcome to *10-Minute Home Workouts for Seniors!*

> **A 2021 study in the <u>Journal of Musculoskeletal and Neuron Interactions</u> found that seniors who did regular strength training and exercise experienced significant improvements in bone density, heart health, muscle strength, mobility, stability, and overall physical function. This reduced the risk of falls, injuries, and chronic disease.**

If you search online for the famous buzzwords of today – **'Workouts for Seniors'** – you will find thousands of over-explained complicated workout plans and books. Unfortunately, most of these contain too much fluff and are simply not practical to implement into your daily life. However, this book is far different. If you are familiar with my last book – **10-Minute Chair Exercises for Seniors** – you will already know that this is a no-nonsense, straightforward workout book that you can begin to use immediately. The workouts are designed to be as simple as possible to follow, with video demonstrations (page 29), a guided audiobook (to be released), and 1-page summary cutouts of each workout, so you won't have to flip through pages while you exercise.

With that said, if you're eager to get started and have reviewed the safety guidelines and disclaimer, then don't hesitate to jump straight ahead to the first workout! However, if you're new to this and want to learn more about this book and how to easily incorporate the workouts into your daily routine, then keep reading. You'll gain a deeper understanding of what this book has to offer and how it can help you achieve your fitness goals in a practical and sustainable way.

So you want to kickstart your fitness journey and begin feeling healthier without too much hassle? Well, you're in luck! Even if you're someone in your forties or fifties and feeling a bit stagnant, this book is the perfect starting point. The exercises are easy to follow, with clear illustrations and instructions. Plus, there's a unique workout for every day of the week that you can easily do from the comfort of your own home – no equipment needed! With a huge variety to choose from, such are cardio HIIT sessions, core workouts, upper and lower body strength training, and more. It won't be long before you start feeling stronger and more energetic throughout your day.

Don't let the misconception fool you that home workouts are ineffective - these exercises can be pretty tough and challenging! I can vouch for this from personal experience, as well as from testing them out on my senior family members. Plus – as you progress, you can up the ante and make each exercise more difficult. Likewise, if you are finding any exercise too challenging, you can always reduce the reps or effort required.

Now, I won't go into exhaustive detail about the benefits of regular exercise and core workouts - I'm sure you already know the importance of staying active and the risks of being sedentary. After all, I'm sure there was a time in your youth when you were in peak physical condition, participating in sports teams, going on hikes, and running 10k races. However, if you're interested, the next chapter provides further insight into the myriad benefits of exercising as you age. To sum it up, consistent physical activity can potentially help boost your energy levels, lower your blood pressure, and prevent falls and injuries. Maintaining a strong core and a healthy heart becomes even more crucial as you age. And the benefits don't end there - your mental and emotional well-being can also greatly improve.

My name is Brian Hardy, and I am a sports and fitness enthusiast who has been active all my life. I've played football, basketball, athletics, and amateur boxing and have tried my hand at every sport under the sun. My fitness regimen over the years has included yoga, deep stretching and mobility work, Pilates, strength training, cross-fit, and HIIT (high-intensity-interval-training). There's not a workout out there that I haven't tried myself.

I currently coach high school and local sports teams, along with studying sports psychology and strength and conditioning. Over my career, I've had numerous fitness issues and injuries—particularly lower back pain. So, I've done extensive personal research in this area.

Once again, for this book, I have teamed up with my good friend and colleague Michael Sheehan, a qualified chartered physiotherapist who has been working with professional sports teams for over a decade. He has enormous experience working in sports physio rehabilitation centers, helping people of all ages recover from injuries and prevent them in future. Michael has also been running core and mobility workout classes for senior citizens over the years. In these classes, his main focus is to enhance strength, stability, and mobility, recognizing the significance of maintaining a strong core and an active body, particularly as you grow older.

Michael has already helped me with the hugely successful: *'10-Minute Chair Exercises for Seniors'* Book. If you are not familiar with it and are looking for something less taxing on the knees and joints (as it involves all seated exercises), then be sure to check it out!

Here is a link or QR code if you are interested:

Link: *'10-Minute Chair Exercises for Seniors'*

QR code: (scan with your phone camera)

Again, we thrashed out and tested countless exercises and devised 7 simple, 10-minute varied workouts, one for every day of the week. Michael has approved every workout, which contains 10 different exercises. The workouts included are as follows:

- **Standard Warm-Up** – This is a series of stretches and movements to loosen out all the joints and get the body moving and warmed up. It's recommended to do this warm-up before any workout.

- **Monday** – **Upper Body Strength Day** – A number of exercises to strengthen all the upper body muscles such as shoulders, biceps, chest, back muscles, and more.

- **Tuesday** – **Cardio HIIT Session 1** – A **H**igh-**I**ntensity **I**nterval **T**raining session where you will perform each exercise for 30 seconds, with a rest of 30 seconds after each one.

- **Wednesday** – **Back Release Stretching** - A stretching session focused on releasing the muscles in your back to help relieve any stiffness.

- **Thursday** – **Core Strength Day** - A core strengthening workout for the abdominal muscles, which are crucial for everyday activities.

- **Friday** – **Lower Body Strength Day** – A number of exercises to strengthen all leg muscles such as Hamstrings, calves, quads, glutes, and more.

- **Saturday** – **Cardio Boxing HIIT Session 2** - A boxing-themed workout that encompasses a variety of boxing exercises and movement – with 30 seconds of work followed by 30 seconds of rest.

- **<u>Sunday</u> – Yoga** - A relaxing but challenging yoga session focused on breathing, stretching, relieving tension, and core strengthening.

Difficulty Levels 1 & 2

I have divided this workout book into two levels of difficulty. I strongly recommend that you start with level 1 and progress to level 2 only after you feel comfortable and can complete the routines with ease. Whether that takes you 3 weeks or 3 months, it does not matter. Just don't jump the gun too soon! Read the chapter on **"How to Use this Book** for more information on the different levels.

Most of the exercises in this book combine elements of core, cardio, and stretching. Proper stretching involves engaging your core, and having good form (technique) during cardio requires flexibility and core engagement. So is important to understand that all elements overlap in a well-rounded workout routine.

No Equipment Needed

Aside from using a chair or wall for balance, and a couple of bottles of water or cans, there really is no equipment needed to do these workouts! Yes, technically you could say, *'But I need a chair'* but in all honestly you can use anything for balance. The same goes for the upper body workouts– you can use cans of food, bottles of water, or anything that weighs a KG or 2. There is one other exercise called step-ups – you can use a small stand or the first step of the stairs – anything that gives you a small bit of height. But that's it, every other exercise does not need equipment! No barbells, no resistant bands, no medicine balls, nothing of the sort, thankfully

In the upcoming chapter, ***The Importance of Exercise for Seniors,*** I will elaborate on the potential benefits of home workouts, such as cardio, stretching, yoga, and core strengthening. This chapter will also detail the potential mental and emotional benefits of regular exercise, so I strongly recommend that you read through it if you haven't already.

The final chapter explains how to get the best out of this book and how to integrate the workouts into your daily routine. Starting a workout routine may seem daunting, but after a few weeks of doing these routines, you may notice significant improvements in energy levels and strength. As a result, you may experience a better quality of life overall. So have fun, and I hope you enjoy the workouts!

THE IMPORTANCE OF EXERCISE FOR SENIORS

As we get older, our bodies go through several changes. As a senior citizen, it's important to understand how the typical aging process works and identify activities that can help prevent injuries, boost your overall health, and enhance your quality of life. In the following section, we'll explore the advantages of exercise and physical activity during senior years. We'll also emphasize the significance of the body's core and suggest different low-impact activities, including stretching and yoga, that are beneficial for seniors and that can be performed at home.

Benefits of Exercise
Ensuring to get regular exercise every week is of utmost importance for a senior's health and well-being. Engaging in physical activity on a regular basis can significantly enhance your overall wellness, including physical, mental, and emotional health. Sedentary lifestyles have been linked to an increased risk of developing chronic diseases such as diabetes, heart disease, and obesity. Therefore, increasing your activity level

can reduce the likelihood of chronic conditions and help you maintain a healthy weight and BMI (**B**ody **M**ass **I**ndex). Consistent exercise has also been shown in research to positively affect mental health, by helping reduce stress levels and improve overall mood. In addition, it can enhance your stamina, fitness, and strength, thereby increasing energy levels and reducing feelings of fatigue. Aerobic activities have been found to activate and strengthen the immune system, decreasing the chances of developing viral illnesses. By prioritizing regular exercise, seniors can help significantly improve their overall health and quality of life.

Significance of Aerobic Activity

Cardiovascular activity, or aerobic exercise, is a crucial component of a healthy lifestyle, especially as the body ages. Often referred to as simply *'cardio* – It can offer numerous potential health benefits to seniors, particularly regarding their cardiovascular (heart) health. Regular aerobic exercise has been shown to positively impact plasma lipids, also known as cholesterol. Specifically, it reduces the levels of low-density lipoprotein (LDL), commonly referred to as "bad cholesterol," while increasing the levels of high-density lipoprotein (HDL), or "good cholesterol" Moreover, this type of exercise helps lower blood pressure and strengthens the heart's pumping ability, allowing it to circulate blood more effectively throughout the body. As a result, you may experience increased energy levels and an improved mood.

Strengthening Exercises – Upper and Lower Body

Growing older naturally leads to a decline in strength and overall physical function. This is due to reduced physical activity, changes in hormones, and the natural aging process. But regular exercise, particularly strengthening exercises, can help slow down or even reverse this decline.

Investing in upper and lower body strengthening exercises can help maintain or improve muscle strength, along with enhancing balance, stability, and mobility. Another crucial benefit is that they help seniors maintain their independence. Falls and injuries increase as we get older. This affects simple daily activities. But by maintaining or improving muscle strength, seniors can reduce the risk of falls and easily perform tasks such as carrying groceries and walking up the stairs. By exercising the legs, hips, and core muscles, seniors can improve their balance and reduce the risk of falling.

Strengthening exercises can also help to **reduce joint pain**, especially in the knees, hips, and shoulders. Strengthening the muscles around these joints can improve mobility and relieve pain. On top of this, they can also maintain or improve bone density, which is essential in preventing fractures and maintaining overall health.

Using resistance bands, dumbbells, and bodyweight exercises are all effective ways to build muscle strength. Exercises include lunges, squats, push-ups, shoulder presses, and much more. Again, always consult with your healthcare provider before starting a new routine. Start slowly and gradually increase the intensity of the workouts over time. It's recommended to do strengthening exercises once or twice per week, with a focus on working all major muscle groups.

The Importance of your Core

The term "core" is commonly used to refer to the central part of the body, which is also known as the abdomen. However, this is an oversimplification. In reality, the core is comprised of a group of muscles that stabilize and control the pelvis and spine. These muscles are responsible for providing support to the body and are essential for performing basic daily activities, such as sitting with an upright posture, moving from one chair or position to another, and showering, to name a few. As we age, getting out of bed and picking things up off the floor can become more challenging, and without a strong core, there is a heightened risk of back injuries.

Additionally, the core is engaged when standing, interacting with family members, and playing with your grandchildren. Seniors can engage and strengthen their core through a variety of exercises, which can easily be done at home.

When the core muscles are strong and working together, they improve balance and stability, which can enhance overall wellness. Specifically, having a strong core can result in better posture, increased flexibility, improved balance, less back pain, and a decreased risk of falls. A strong core can also help ensure proper form and technique during exercise.

The Downside of a Weak Core

Regrettably, neglecting activities that promote core strength can lead to a weakened core, which in turn increases the risk of injuries and pain. A weak core can lead to an elevated risk of lower back pain and discomfort, as well as reduced flexibility and stability for seniors. Consequently, maintaining an upright posture and balance may become difficult for seniors, resulting in an increased likelihood of falls and injuries. These injuries can be severe and may take weeks or more to recover from. A weakened core can also impede your ability to transfer from one chair or position to another, making it challenging to perform basic daily activities and potentially impacting your quality of life.

The Value of Stretching

Stretching is an important daily activity for seniors that helps to increase flexibility by lengthening the muscles. This is especially beneficial as the body ages since muscles tend to shorten naturally and become tighter without regular stretching. Tight muscles can increase the risk of injuries. Stretching helps to make these muscles more flexible and allows for a fuller range of motion in the joints, again decreasing the likelihood of discomfort and injury. Furthermore, stretching improves blood flow to the muscles, enabling them to work more effectively. There are numerous stretches that seniors can do to stretch their muscles in a healthy and beneficial way. Overall, stretching will help to leave you feeling looser and able to perform basic activities with less effort.

Benefits of Yoga

Yoga is another excellent form of stretching and exercise for seniors that has many benefits for both the mind and body. The word "yoga" comes from the Sanskrit language and means "union" or "yoke." It is a spiritual practice that dates back centuries and is designed to bring together the body, mind, and spirit. Practicing yoga regularly can help to promote good health, both physically and mentally. There are many different types of yoga, but all emphasize the importance of posture, breathing, and meditation.

In today's world, all forms of yoga are accessible to people of all ages and fitness levels. Although some styles may be more challenging, modifications can always be made to accommodate seniors or beginners. Thanks to the internet, guided Yoga sessions can be done from the comfort of your home whenever you feel like it.

There are numerous potential health benefits to be gained from practicing yoga regularly. One of the key advantages is that it involves working a variety of muscle groups through controlled movements and prolonged holding postures. This can improve muscle strength and flexibility, as well as increase blood flow to the muscles. Yoga breathing techniques can also be used to manage stress levels, which can help reduce inflammation. In addition to these physical benefits, yoga can also greatly improve your overall mental and emotional health. This often happens as a result of learning new yoga techniques for coping with anxiety and depression. Some findings suggest yoga practices can also enhance balance and promote better sleep. The emphasis on correct posture in yoga by using and engaging the core muscles also helps to reduce lower back pain and improve stability. Overall, regular yoga practice can contribute to improved flexibility, wellness, and overall physical and mental health.

Conclusion

There are countless reasons why exercise is vital for maintaining good physical health, especially for seniors. While there are no claims or guarantees, it's entirely possible that by establishing a regular exercise routine, seniors can improve their heart health, and improve their mental and emotional well-being by managing stress levels. Remember, you want to be active and pain-free for as long as possible, and this, in turn, will improve and maintain a good quality of life.

Although starting a new exercise routine can be challenging, it is important to take the initiative and begin to experience the numerous benefits that come with it. Those benefits will soon outweigh any doubts and resistance you initially had to working out. In this book, you now have a variety of strengthening, stretching, cardio, and core workout routines that can be done any time in the comfort of your home. There's no time like the present to begin a new journey!

HOW TO USE THIS BOOK

This section includes some helpful tips on how to make the most of this book. First of all, be sure to look through the exercises of each workout before you begin so you understand how to do each one correctly. I intentionally made the steps provided with each illustration short and easy to follow without being too detailed.

Take the time to read the introduction to each workout, which will tell you what type of workout it is and how to get started in the comfort of your own home. The video demonstrations will be linked via a **_QR code_** at the end of this chapter. Simply scan the QR code with your phone, and it will take you straight to the video demos. If there are any illustrations you still need clarification on, please watch the video demonstrations for a more precise idea. Please note that the videos are not timed to the correct number of reps or second holds for each exercise. They are purely for demonstration and technique purposes.

Remember to drink a glass of water before working out. It's important to read over the safety disclaimer and always warm up correctly before you start each workout. Don't push yourself too hard, especially if you are feeling unwell.

Lastly, I have included a cut-out summary page for each workout. I recommend you cut this page out with a scissors and ask a friend or family member who works in a school or an office to laminate it for you. After doing the workouts a few times, you will be familiar with the exercises and names of each one, so you won't have to flip through the pages and can glance at the summary page cut-out instead to guide you.

Workout Logs

At the beginning of this book, you'll find a link or QR code that will lead you to a printable progress tracker logbook that you can download. The best way to use this logbook is to simply put an X on the days that you work out. This method, which I learned from James Clear, author of 'Atomic Habits,' is an extremely effective way to reinforce the habit you're trying to develop by giving you a hit of dopamine as you see the X's accumulate. I've even used this myself, marking an X for every day I did a 5k run or did one hour of writing. You'll find yourself wanting to add more to the logbook without even realizing it, and eventually, you won't be able to stand seeing too many blank spaces, ensuring you have more Xs than blanks. You can use this logbook for any goal or daily habit you want to establish.

The logbook is divided into 4-week blocks. If you've done 4 or 5 workouts a week for four weeks, taking a rest week could be a good idea. Listen to your body and decide how you're feeling. If you feel better than ever and want to keep going, then by all means do that! Always assess your energy levels and trust your intuition.

It's also not vital that you complete the specific workout on that particular day. If, for example, you're feeling great benefits from the core workout and want to do it again on Monday, that's great! A good idea would be to add 'CO' or 'HT' beside the X to indicate whether it was a core workout or a cardio HIIT workout.

As a guideline, if you're doing three workouts a week, aim for one cardio, one core or strengthening, and one stretching or yoga. Keep it simple, build up your Xs, and soon you'll be proud of how much progress you've made, and it will motivate you even more!

Pay attention to your workout balance. If you're overloading on one type of workout and neglecting another, just make sure to balance it out in the following weeks. You can always mix in the chair workouts if you are already familiar with those from the previous workout program.

Free Audiobook Guide

This workout book will come with a complimentary audiobook guide that will provide a guided narration for each workout, with background workout music included. This audiobook should be ready in the coming months and will be sent straight to you free of charge. To access this free audiobook, click on the link or QR code at the beginning of the book, the same one you use for the Workout logbook download. The audio guide will be timed to allow time for each exercise and will ensure you spend the correct amount of time on each one. For example, the cardio HIIT sessions are timed at 30-second intervals, so you won't have to worry about having a stopwatch. A beeper will be played for you. For the other workouts, reps will be counted, or enough time will be left for you to complete them. Everything is in place to make these workouts as simple as possible, and enjoyable!

Difficulty Levels 1 and 2

You should start at Difficulty Level 1, which includes the Standard Warm-Up and the 7 daily workouts from Monday to Sunday. Difficulty Level 2 contains the very same workouts, this time with increased effort and difficulty.

For example, the Cardio HIIT sessions in Level 2 will increase to 35 seconds of work with 25 seconds rest, or if you want to make it even harder – 40 seconds on with 20 seconds rest. This will be a lot more exerting that Difficulty Level 1 – 30 seconds of work with 30 seconds rest. Although it might not seem like a big jump, those extra 5 seconds of work and 5 seconds less rest will make a big impact!

For the core and strengthening workouts, you will be doing an increased number of REPS in level 2 compared to level 1. The stretching and yoga sessions remain the same. It is essential that you **DO NOT SKIP TO LEVEL 2 TOO SOON –** only do so when you find level 1 becomes too easy. For some people, this may only take 4 or 5 weeks. But for the average individual, it could take months or longer. What matters most is that you are working out regularly and enjoying yourself, not how long it takes to progress. By working out regularly, you are already doing more than most people your age – so you are already on the winning team.

It's important to note that for some people, level 1 can be challenging enough. If you find it tough to complete a cardio session, you don't have to work for the full 30 seconds recommended. Aim to get to 15 or 20 seconds of work instead, and this will give you added time to recover between rounds. Over time, you can gradually build up to the 30-second mark. This goes for the number of REPS and hold times in other exercises also. Do as many as you can, and build up the numbers week after week.

Lastly, it is not the end of the world if you miss a workout from time to time. It's also not crucial that you follow the specific workout for each day. If you are suffering from stiffness in your back and it's Monday, by all means go ahead and do the 'Wednesday back release stretching session or the 'Sunday yoga session. Likewise, If you are enjoying the cardio workouts, then feel free to do them on whatever days you please. Personally, I think the best thing is to do these workouts sometime in the morning. Then you have the whole day ahead of you, and you can feel a sense of satisfaction knowing you have got some physical activity in, which can lead to a healthier lifestyle.

The goal of this book is to get you back moving. Even if you go from being inactive to just doing a couple of workouts a week, that's something to be proud of! You can then gradually increase the number of workouts as your energy levels increase. Remember, just 10 minutes can have a tremendous positive impact on your life. Enjoy your workouts!

VIDEOS DEMONSTRATIONS

FOR WORKOUTS

To access the workout video demonstrations, just scan the **QR code** below with your phone camera. It will take you to every workout demonstration video for each day:

QR Code:

As I mentioned earlier, the exercises are **not performed to the appropriate length of time or the correct number of reps.** They are purely for demonstration purposes in case you still don't fully understand the illustrations and steps.

(Always make sure to read the introduction section of each workout carefully – along with the Health and Safety disclaimer at the beginning of the book, before starting your exercises)

LEVEL 1

1.0 - STANDARD WARM-UP

1.0 – STANDARD WARM-UP

Welcome to your standard warm-up! This warm-up contains 10 simple stretches and exercises to warm up your muscles and get the blood flowing. By doing the given routine, your joints will be loosened up, and you will be ready to work out and push your body outside its comfort zone. It's essential you do this full standard warm-up before every workout. This warm-up contains the following:

- Loosening your **shoulders**, **spine,** and other joint areas
- **Stretching** your upper body and lower body muscles
- **Loosening** out any stiff areas
- And more…

It is advised to use the **Free Audiobook** (once released) as a guide for these workouts, as it is timed and guides you through each exercise.

Please check the video demonstrations using the **QR code on page 29** for the correct form and technique. After some time, these exercises will become second nature, and you will instantly know what to do.

Have a good warm-up!

1 SHAKE IT OUT

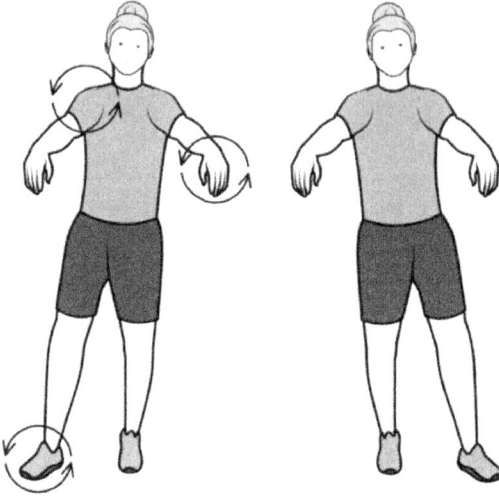

15+ Seconds

- shake / loosen arms + legs

2 SHOULDER ROTATIONS

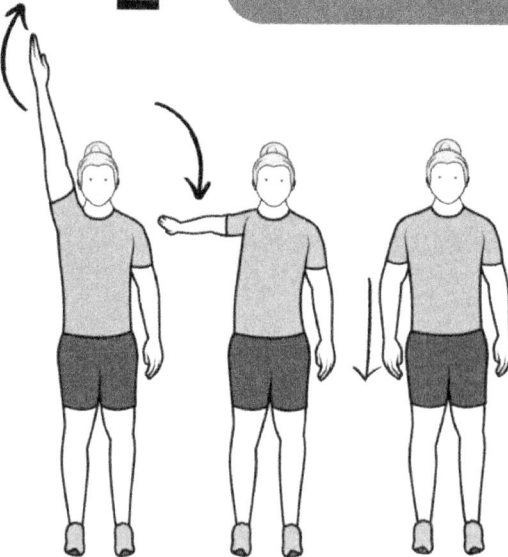

X3 each side

- full rotations around and back around on each arm

- (see video demo)

3 CROSS ARM STRETCH

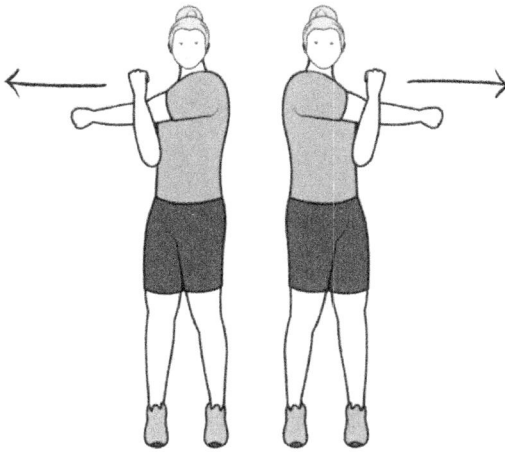

X2 each side

- cross arm across chest

- 5-second holds each side

4 HAMSTRING STRETCH

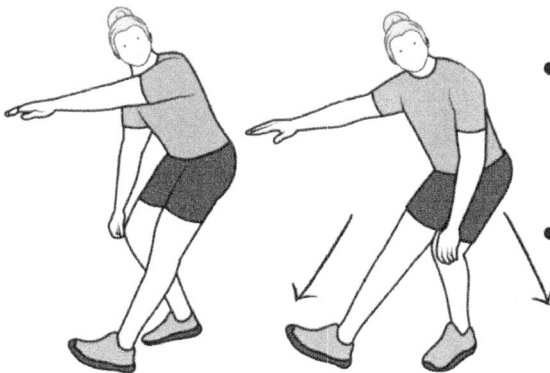

X3 each side

- 5-second holds on each leg

- Sit back - lock out leg - toe facing up - hand out

5   GROIN STRETCH

X3 each side

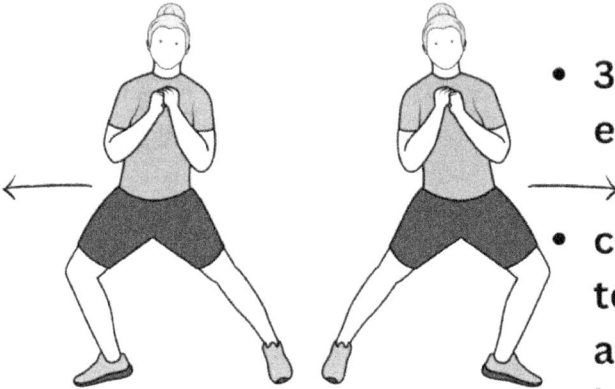

- 3-second holds each side

- core engaged, toe pointing away on bent leg

6   CALF STRETCH

X2 each side

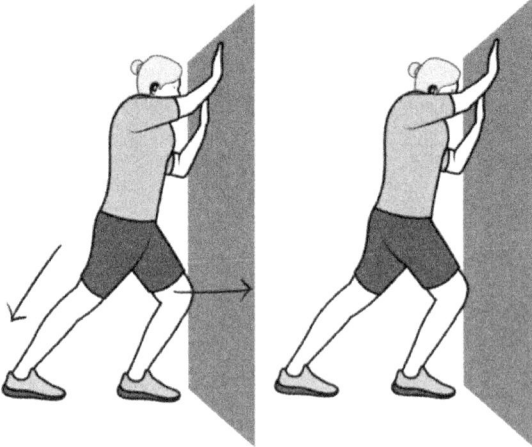

- 10-second hold each leg

- push knee to wall + lock out knee on back leg + heel to ground

7 CHEST ROTATIONS

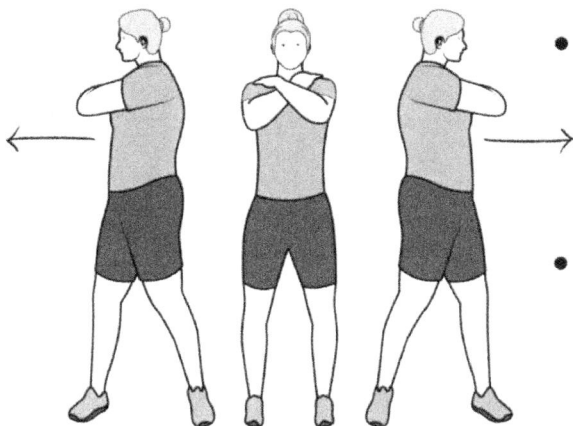

X3 each side

- cross arms + rotate upper body

- (5 second hold on each twist - back straight + core engaged)

8 REACH UP -> TOE TOUCH

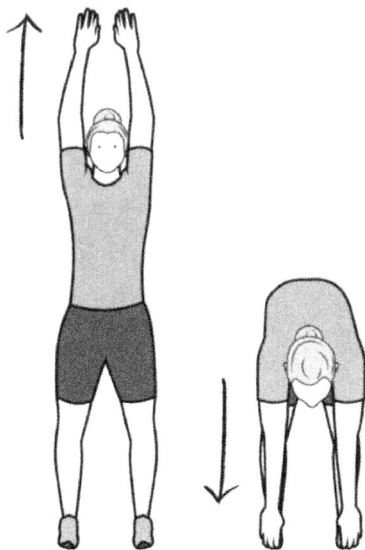

X2

- reach tall as possible on tippy toes

  +

- fold down slowly and touch your shin/toes

9 RUNNING ON THE SPOT

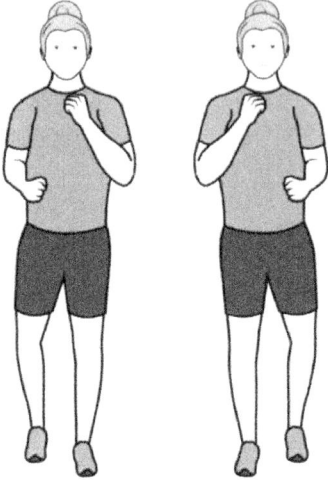

15+ seconds

- jogging on the spot

10 SHAKE IT OUT

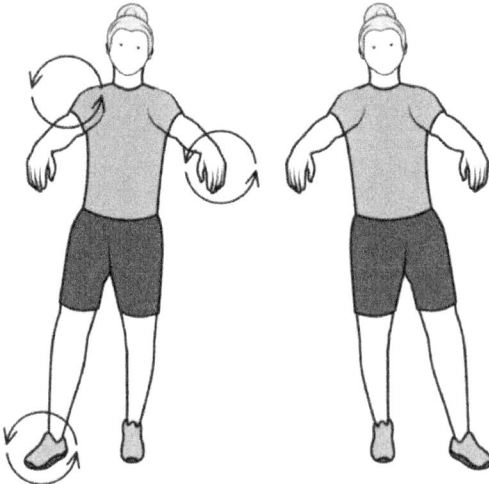

15+ Seconds

- shake / loosen arms + legs

1.0 - WARM-UP SUMMARY

1 SHAKE IT OUT

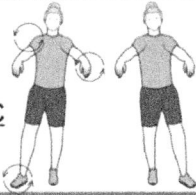

15+ SEC

2 SHOULDER ROTATIONS

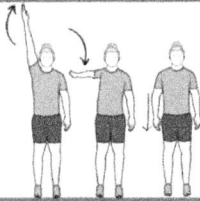

X3 ES

3 CROSS ARM STRETCH

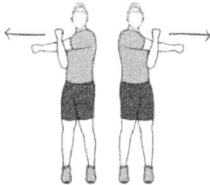

X2 ES

4 HAMSTRING STRETCH

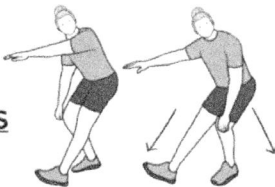

X3 ES

5 GROIN STRETCH

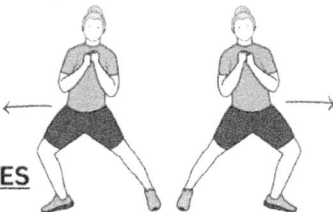

X3 ES

6 CALF STRETCH

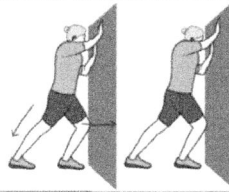

X2 ES

7 CHEST ROTATIONS

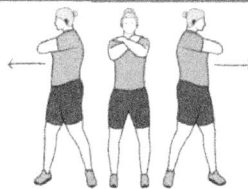

X3 ES

8 REACH UP -> TOE TOUCH

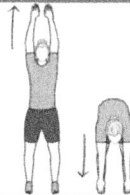

X2

9 RUNNING ON THE SPOT

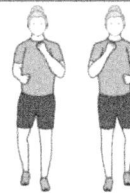

15+ SEC

10 SHAKE IT OUT

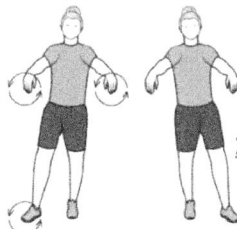

15+ SEC

BRIAN HARDY

1.1 - MONDAY - UPPER BODY STRENGTH

1.1 – MONDAY – UPPER BODY

Welcome to **Monday's Upper Body Strength** Day! Be sure to drink plenty of water and warm up correctly before starting. This workout contains several upper-body exercises such as:

- **Bicep, tricep,** and **shoulder** exercises
- **Back** and **chest** exercises
- **Stability** exercises using your **core muscles** for correct form and technique

There are 10 varying exercises with a number of reps to complete for each exercise, so it should take a total of 10 minutes to complete. All you need is 2 cans of food, 2 water bottles, or anything that weighs a KG or 2 – That's it!

It is advised to use the **Free Audiobook** (once released) as a guide for these workouts, as it is timed and guides you through each exercise.

Please check the video demonstrations using the **QR code on page 29** for correct form and technique. You should never be in pain doing any exercises. Please ensure correct form by stabilizing your core muscles and keeping a bend on your knees and a straight back.

Have a good workout!

1 WALL PUSH-UPS

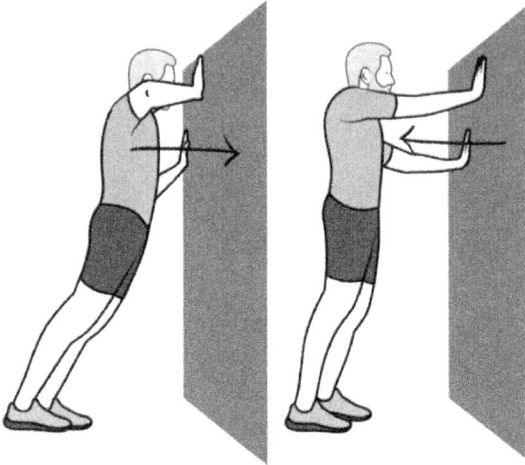

X10

- lean chest close to wall

- push out + lock elbows

2 SHOULDER BLADE SQUEEZES

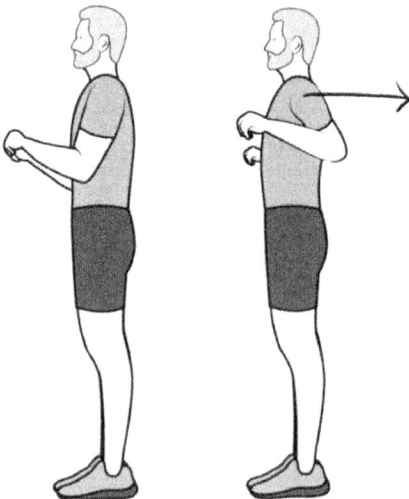

X10
(focus on shoulder blades)

- pull elbows back + squeeze shoulder blades for 3 seconds

3 BICEP CURLS

<u>X10</u>

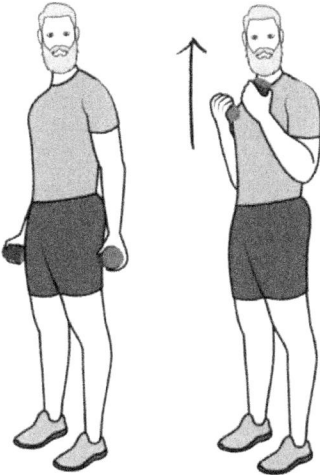

- bend elbows + curl biceps up and down

(use cans of food or bottles of water or light dumbbells)

4 BENT OVER ROWS

<u>X10</u>

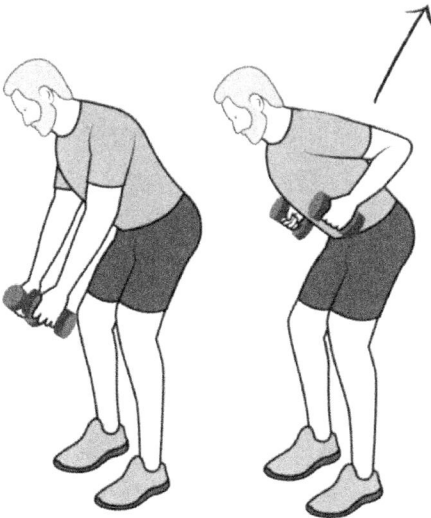

- slight lean forward + bend knees + engage core + straight back

- squeeze shoulder blades + 10 rows with cans/bottles /weights

5 CHEST PRESS

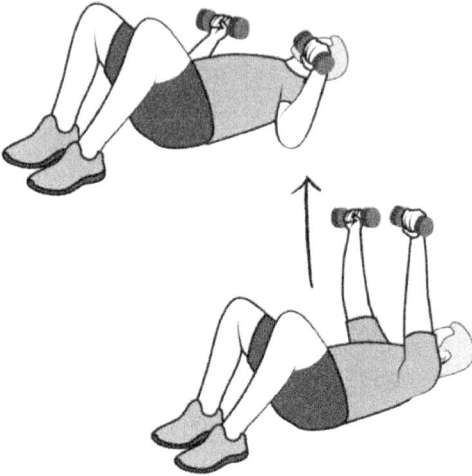

X10

- lie down on floor + bend knees

- bend elbows to touch floor then press up straight and down

6 TRICEP EXTENSIONS

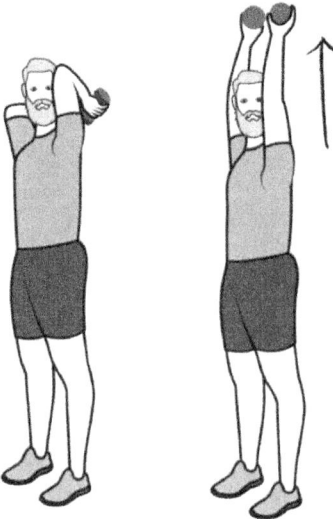

X10

- hold cans/bottles behind head as shown, bend elbows then extend up using triceps

- (engage core + straight back)

7 SHOULDER PRESS

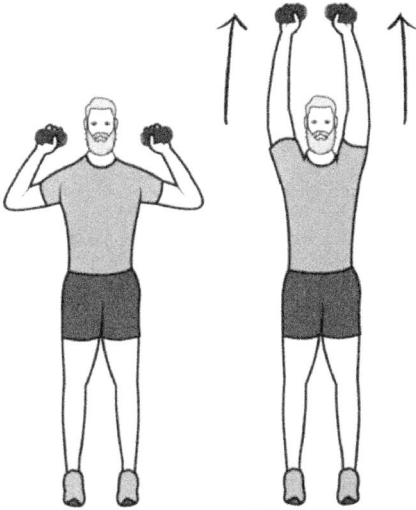

X10

- hold cans/bottles to side of head as shown + extend overhead locking arms up

- (engage core + straight back)

8 CHEST FLYS

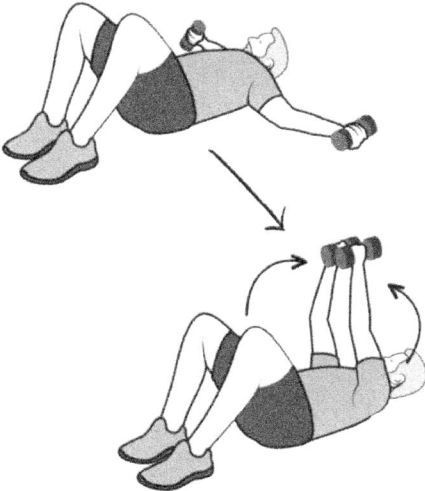

X10

- (lie down on floor + bend knees)

- hold cans straight out touching the ground as shown

- press cans together keeping arms straight

9 REVERSE FLYS

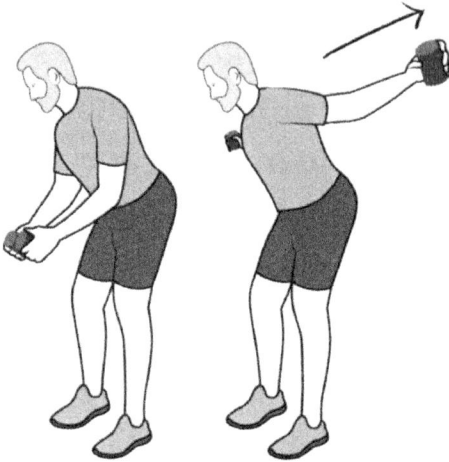

X10
- slight lean forward + bend knees + engage core + straight back
- squeeze shoulder blades + fly back cans as shown + keep arms straight

10 SHOULDER RAISES

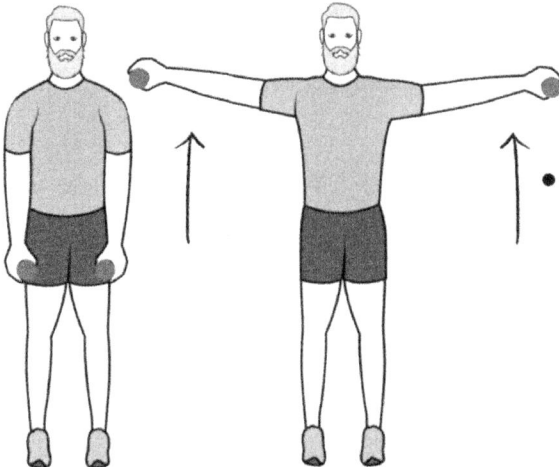

X10
- raise cans up and down with arms straight out to the side using shoulder strength

1.1 – MONDAY – UPPER BODY SUMMARY

1 WALL PUSH-UPS

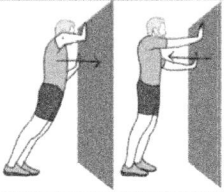

X10

2 SHOULDER BLADE SQUEEZES

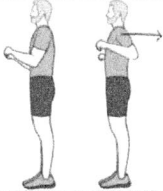

X10

3 BICEP CURLS

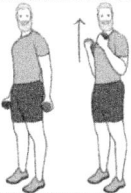

X10

4 BENT OVER ROWS

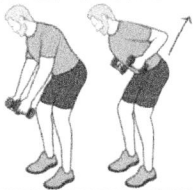

X10

5 CHEST PRESS

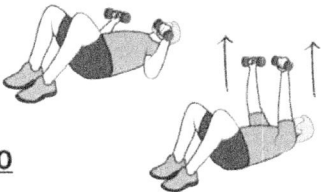

X10

6 TRICEP EXTENSIONS

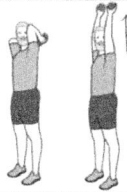

X10

7 SHOULDER PRESS

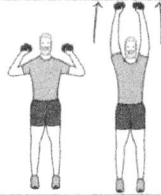

X10

8 CHEST FLYS

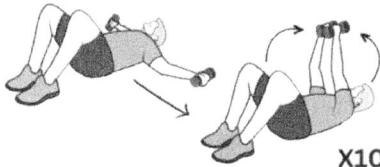

X10

9 REVERSE FLYS

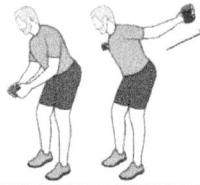

X10

10 SHOULDER RAISES

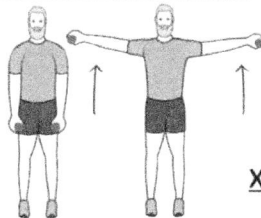

X10

1.2 - TUESDAY - CARDIO HIIT 1

1.2 – TUESDAY – CARDIO HIIT 1

Welcome to **Tuesday's Cardio HIIT** session number 1 of the week! Be sure to drink plenty of water and warm up correctly before starting. This workout will be timed at intervals. As a High-Intensity Interval Training session, this workout will follow this path:

- **30 seconds** of high-intensity work
- Followed by **30 seconds** of rest before beginning the next exercise/round.

There are 10 varying exercises (or rounds), so it should take a total of 10 minutes to complete. You can use the first step of the stairs or a small stand for the step-up exercise.

It is advised to use the **Free Audiobook** (once released) as a guide for these workouts, as it is timed and will tell you when 30 seconds are up for each round. The timer on phones can be awkward as the screen locks, and you cannot see the time.

If you are doing this workout for the first time, it is ok to go at a **medium intensity** for the first few rounds. Slowly over time, you can increase the intensity. You want to push yourself just outside your comfort zone each round. Each week you will notice an improvement.

Please check the video demonstrations using the **QR code on page 29** for the correct form and technique of each exercise.

Have a good workout!

1 **RUNNING ON THE SPOT**

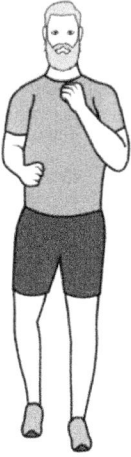 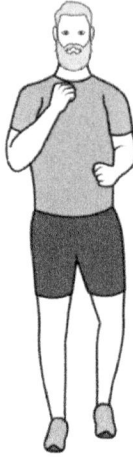

30s on/30s off

- running on the spot

2 **STEP UPS**

30s on/30s off

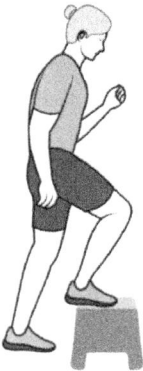 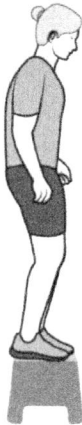 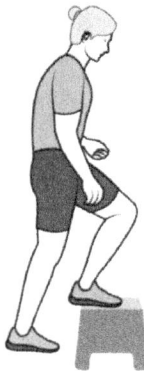

- use box + step up and down quick

- (change stepping foot every 5 steps)

3 CRUNCHES KNEE TO ELBOW

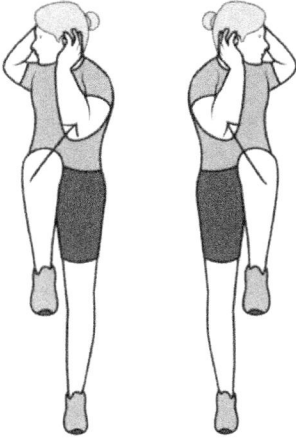

30s on/30s off

- hands to side of head - try touch elbow to opposite knee

- alternate each side

4 PUNCH UP -> PUNCH OUT

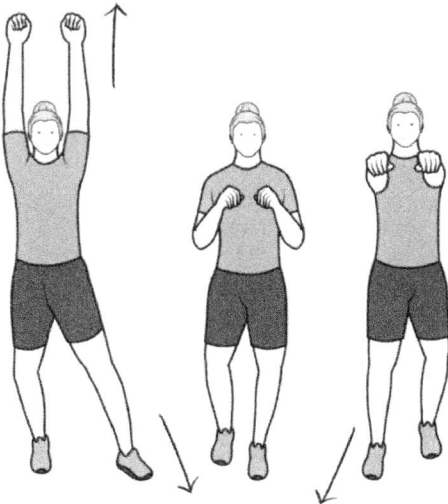

30s on/30s off

- punch up + toe tap to one side

- punch out + toe tap to other side

5 SQUATS

30s on/30s off

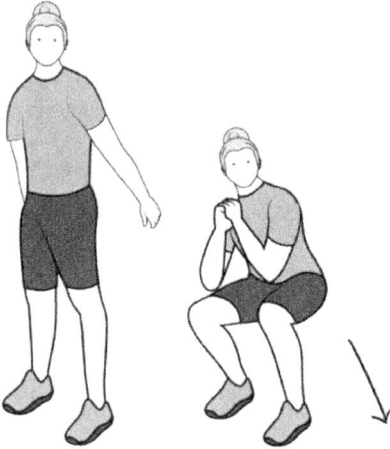

- squat as low as possible then straight back up

- (use a chair to squat on if you need)

6 SIDE STEPS

30s on/30s off

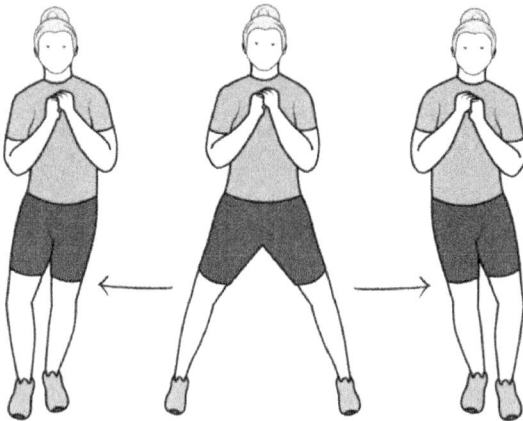

- continuously stepping from side to side

- (see video demo)

7 — LEG CURL AND PRESS

30s on/30s off

- press elbows up and down with triceps + hamstring curls left and right

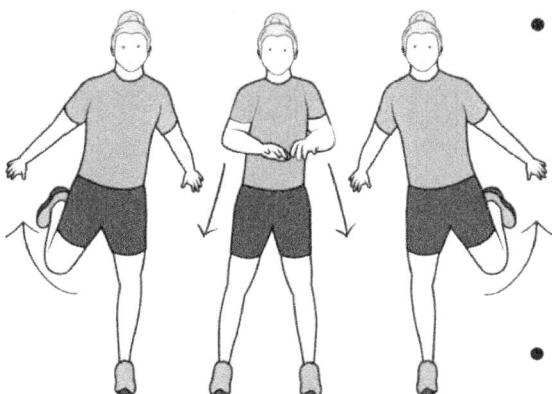

- (see video demo)

8 — PUSH FORWARD AND OUT

30s on/30s off

- push forward + step one side then push out to the side + step to other side -

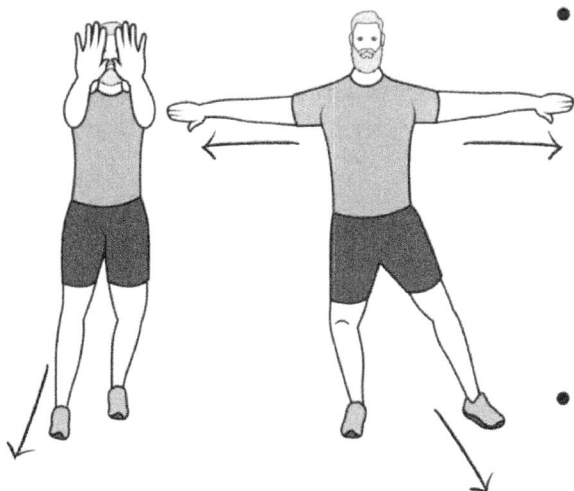

- (see video demo)

9 **JUMPING JACKS**

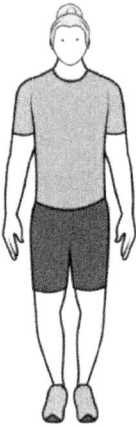

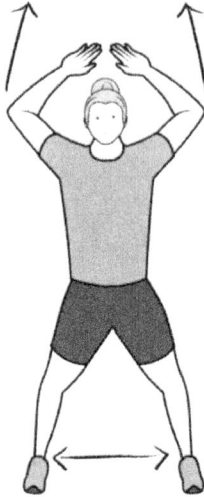

30s on/30s off

- legs out + hands over head

- continuous

10 **RUNNING ON THE SPOT**

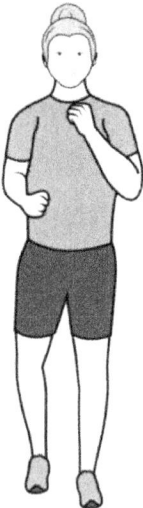

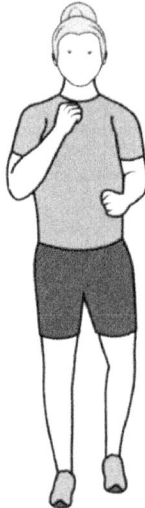

30s on/30s off

- running on the spot at fast pace to finish

1.2 - TUESDAY CARDIO HIIT 1 SUMMARY

1 RUNNING ON THE SPOT

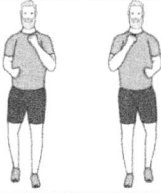

6 SIDE STEPS

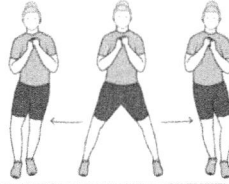

30 SEC WORK | 30 SEC REST

2 STEP-UPS

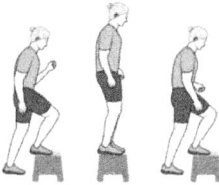

7 LEG CURL AND PRESS

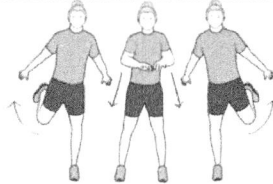

3 CRUNCHES KNEE TO ELBOW

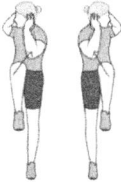

8 PUSH FORWARD AND OUT

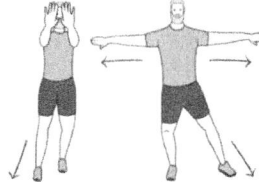

4 PUNCH UP-> PUNCH OUT

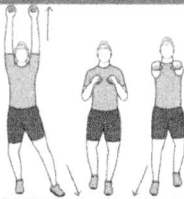

9 JUMPING JACKS

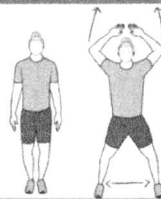

5 SQUATS

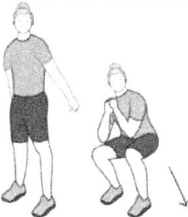

10 RUNNING ON THE SPOT

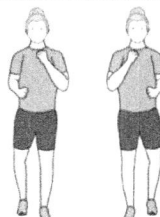

1.3 - WEDNESDAY - BACK RELEASE STRETCHES

1.3 – WEDNESDAY – BACK RELEASE

Welcome to today's **Back Release Stretching** session! Be sure to drink water and warm up correctly before starting. Having a healthy back and spine is crucial to your quality of life. It's all about getting fluid back into your spine and other joints through movement. Today's stretching session will contain the following:

- **Slow and controlled** movements of the joints and spine
- **Engaging your core**
- **Holding deep stretches** in certain positions to release any tension
- And more…

There are 10 **varying** exercises, so it should take approximately 10 minutes to complete. This will be a less intense workout, but keeping a good posture and engaging your core muscles is still crucial. Follow the steps provided. Some exercises will contain timed holds, while others will have repetitions.

It is advised to use the **Free Audiobook** (once released) as a guide for these workouts, as it is timed and guides you through each exercise.

Please check the video demonstrations using the **QR code on page 29** for the correct form and technique of each exercise.

Have a good workout!

1

SHOULDER BLADE ELBOW ROTATIONS

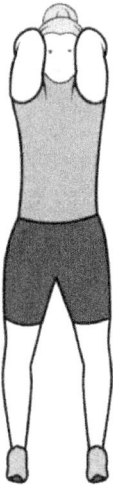

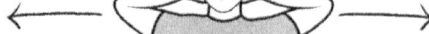

X10

- hands behind head - rotate elbows in and out as shown

- 2 second holds on each rotation

2

HANDS BEHIND HEAD-SIDE TO SIDE

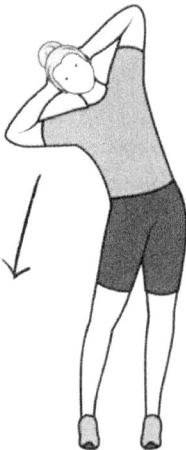

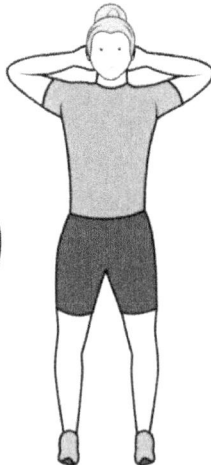

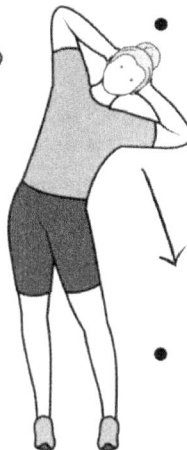

X5 each side

- hands behind head - slowly bend down to side and hold for 3 seconds

- (engage core + straight back)

3 CAT/CAMEL STANDING

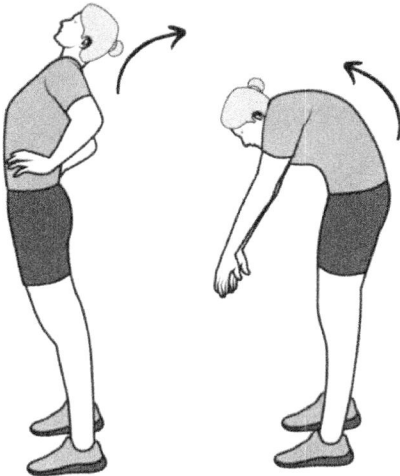

X10

- hand on back, look up + arch back

- change to reach down + round back

- (slow movements)

4 OBLIQUE TWIST AND HOLD

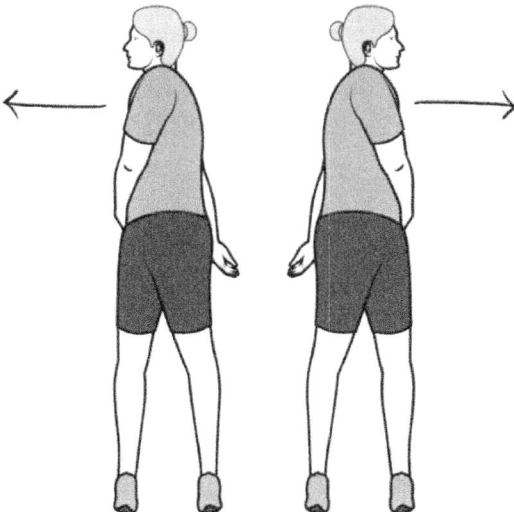

X5 each side

- twist upper body to one side and hold for 5 seconds

5 TALL TO BEND OVER

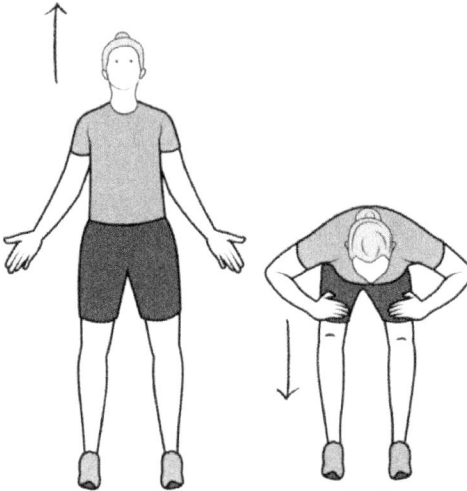

X10
- on tippy toes, stand up tall looking up for 5 seconds

- slowly bend down, hands on legs and hold for 5 seconds

6 SWIMMER REACHES

X10 each side
- wide stance - reach one hand to one side and hold for 2 seconds - change sides

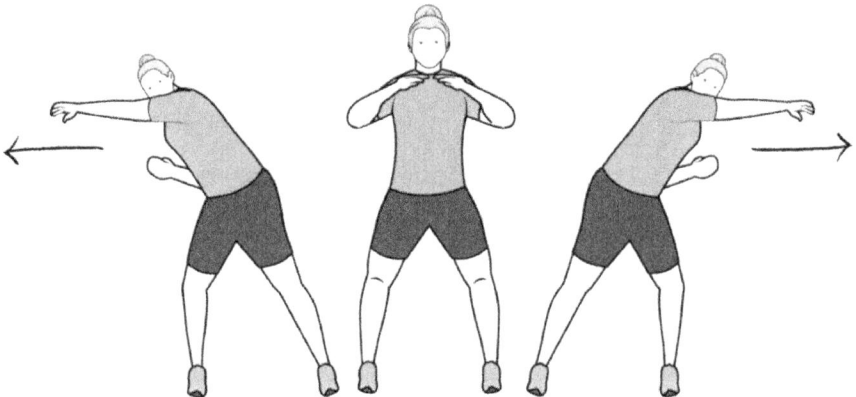

7 STAR SQUAT TO REACH HIGH

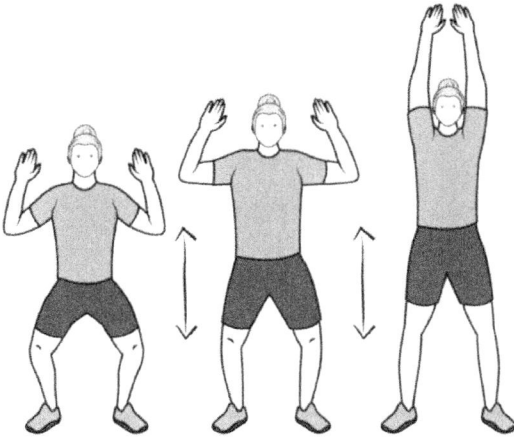

X10
- squat down with hands up as shown

- then squat up + reach hands up

8 ARM CIRCLES

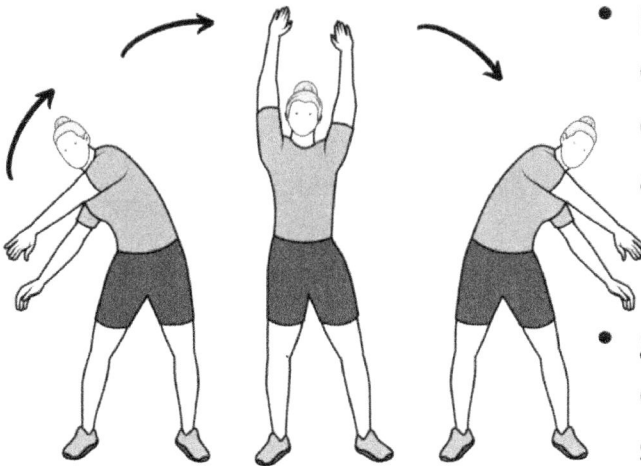

X10 each side
- push hands out + exaggerate arm circles

- go in both directions slowly

9 ROCK TO TALL REACH

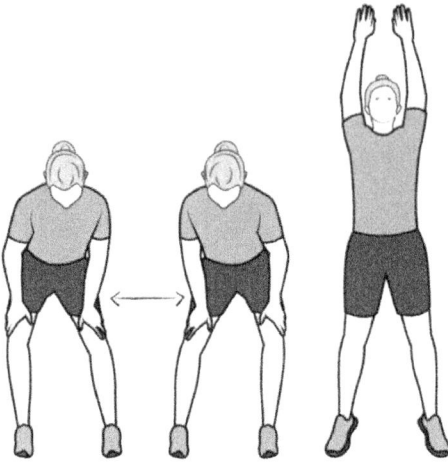

X10

- bend over + rock side to side with hands on legs

- then reach hands tall + reach back

10 UPPERBODY FREESTYLE-SWAY/LOOSEN

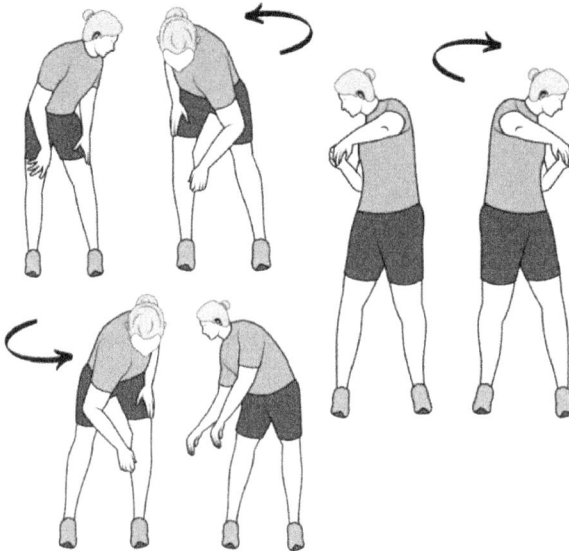

20+ seconds

- freestyle upper-body movements

- (see video demo)

1.3 – WED – BACK RELEASE SUMMARY

1 SHOULDER BLADE ELBOW ROTATIONS

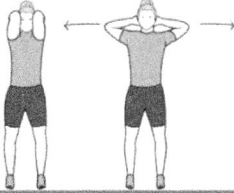

X10

2 HANDS BEHIND HEAD- SIDE TO SIDE

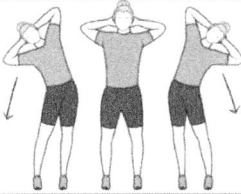

X5 ES

3 CAT/CAMEL STANDING

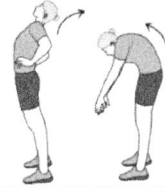

X10

4 OBLIQUE TWIST AND HOLD

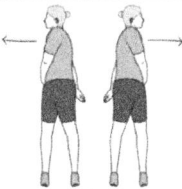

X5 ES

5 TALL TO BEND OVER

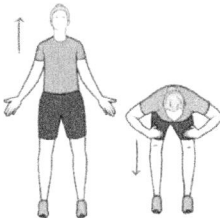

X10

6 SWIMMER REACHES

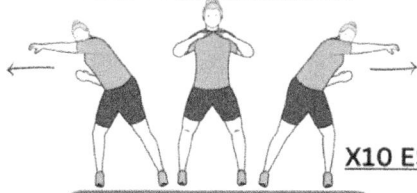

X10 ES

7 STAR SQUAT TO REACH HIGH

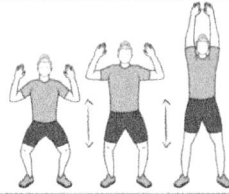

X10

8 ARM CIRCLES

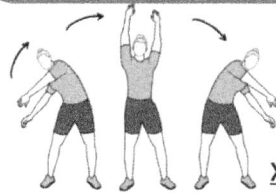

X10 ES

9 ROCK TO TALL REACH

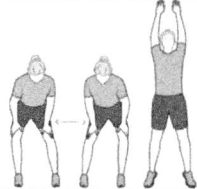

X10

10 UPPER BODY FREESTYLE SWAY/LOOSEN

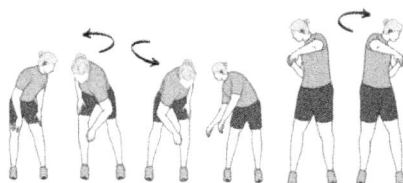

20+ SEC

1.4 - THURSDAY - CORE STRENGTH

1.4 – THURSDAY – CORE STRENGTH

Welcome to today's **Core Strengthening** workout! Be sure to drink water and warm up correctly before starting. With any core workout, it is **vital** you concentrate on **engaging your core** muscles and keeping a **straight back** and **good posture.** This workout will contain the following:

- A variety of **Abdominal** (core) exercises
- Numerous exercises **lying on your back** or **on all fours**
- **Slow and controlled** movements.
- And more…

There are 10 varying exercises, so it should take approximately 10 minutes to complete. If you can feel your core working and burning, you are doing the exercise correctly. If not, then you could be compensating with other parts of your body. So make sure to always engage your core muscles. If you are doing this workout for the first time, go slowly into each movement, and don't go too far outside your comfort zone.

It is advised to use the **Free Audiobook** (once released) as a guide for these workouts, as it is timed and guides you through each exercise.

Please check the video demonstrations using the **QR code on page 29** for the correct form and technique of each exercise.

Have a good workout!

1 SINGLE KNEE CRUNCH

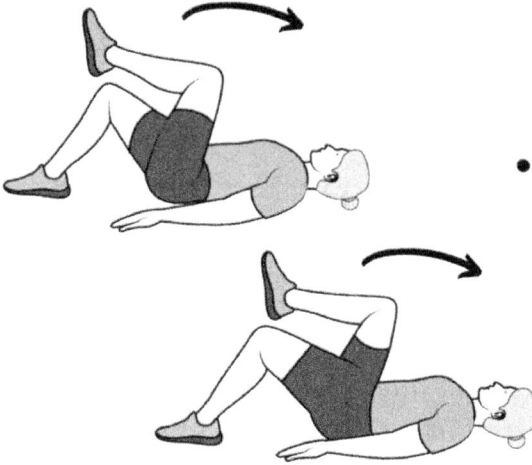

X10 each side

- lie down - arms by side - bend one knee to chest using core

2 DOUBLE KNEE CRUNCH

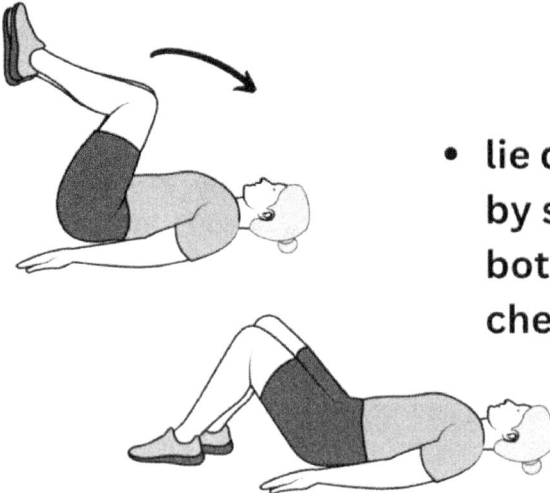

X10

- lie down - arms by side - bend both knees to chest using core

3 KNEE DROPS

X5 each side

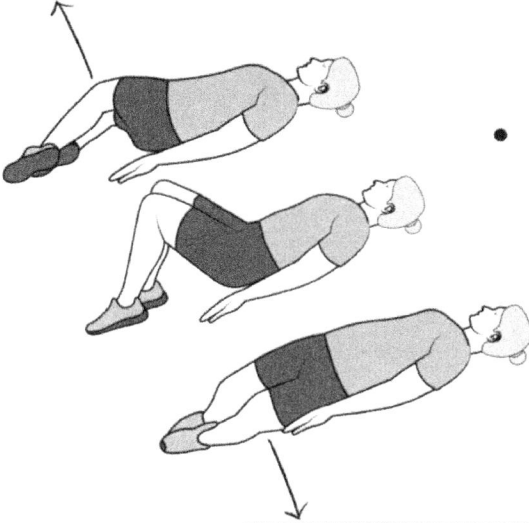

- touch knees + drop them to each side 5 times

4 HEAD CRUNCH UP

X10

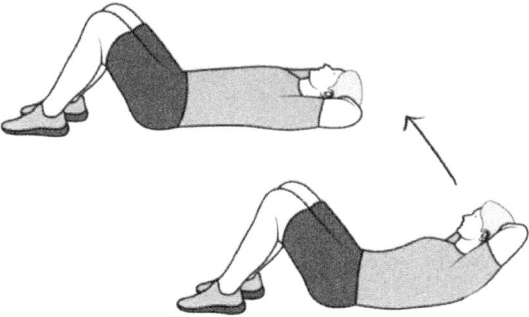

- hands behind head, using core, crunch up

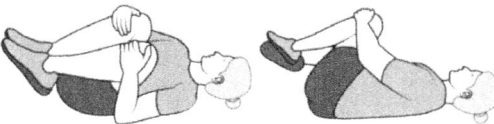

- (Knee hugs + rock for relief after)

5 FULL SINGLE KNEE CRUNCH

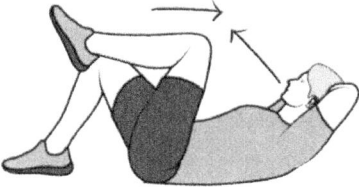

X10 each side

- hands behind head - crunch up with head + crunch one knee to chest

- alternate legs

6 FULL DOUBLE KNEE CURNCH

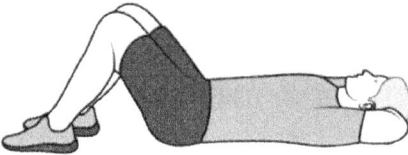

X10

- hands behind head - crunch up with head + crunch both knees to chest

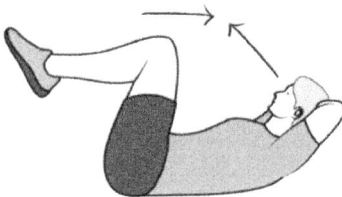

7 HALF DEAD BUG

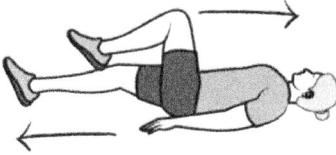

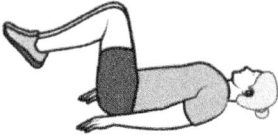

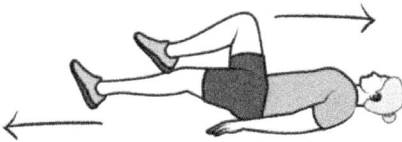

X10 each side
- hands by side - extend one leg out straight + bend other knee up 90 degrees

- change to opposite legs

8 FULL DEAD BUG

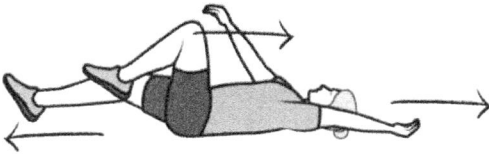

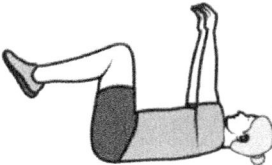

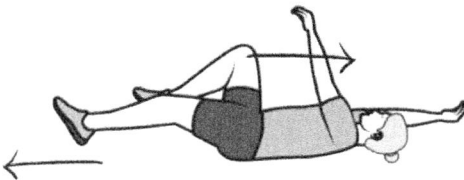

X10
- add in arms - raise arm of bent knee + alternate each side

- (straight leg + opposite straight arm

9 BIRD DOG

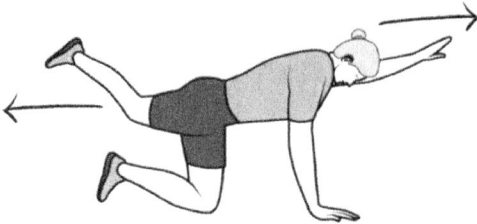

X10 each side

- on all fours - straight left hand out + straight right leg out

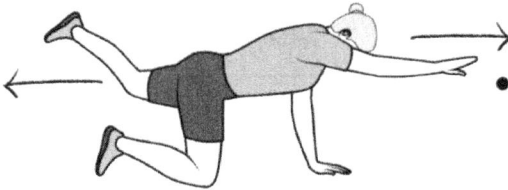

- change + alternate each leg and hand

10 CAT/CAMEL TO CHILDS POSE

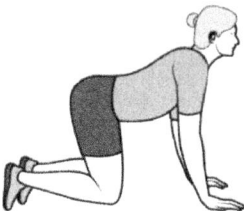

X5

- do the cat + camel pose slowly - then sit into childs pose pushing bum back + arms out in front

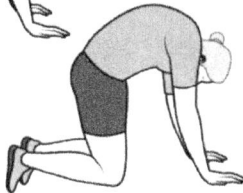

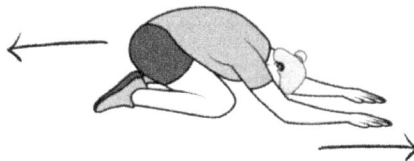

1.4 – THURSDAY – CORE STRENGTH SUMMARY

1 SINGLE KNEE CRUNCH

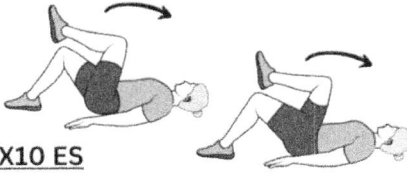

X10 ES

2 DOUBLE KNEE CRUNCH

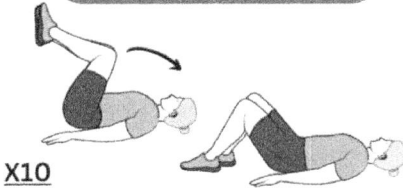

X10

3 KNEE DROPS

X5 ES

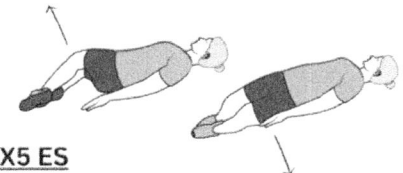

4 HEAD CRUNCH UP (KNEE ROCKS)

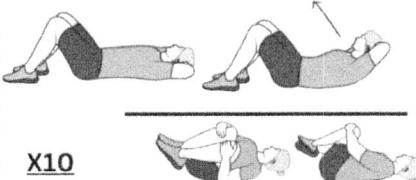

X10

5 FULL SINGLE KNEE CRUNCH

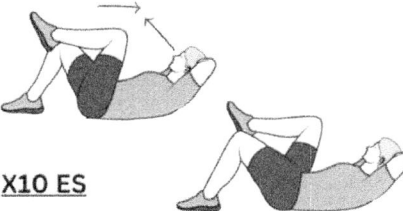

X10 ES

6 FULL DOUBLE KNEE CRUNCH

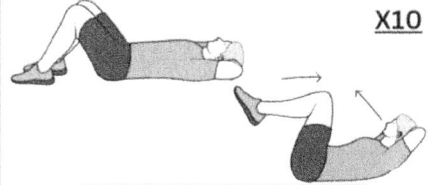

X10

7 HALF DEAD BUG

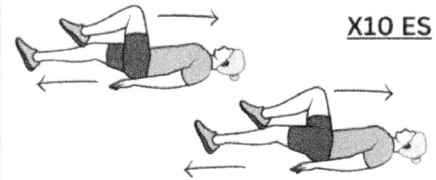

X10 ES

8 FULL DEAD BUG

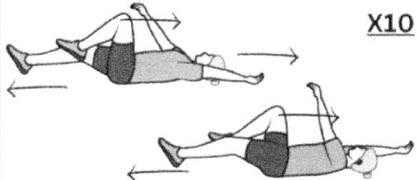

X10

9 BIRD DOG

X10 ES

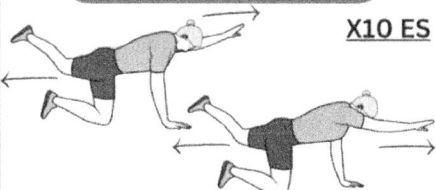

10 CAT/CAMEL TO CHILDS POSE

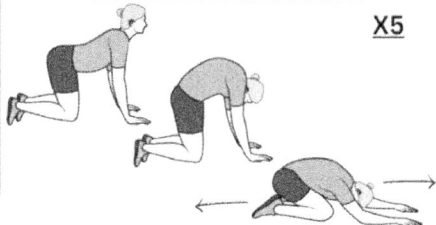

X5

1.5 - FRIDAY - LOWER BODY STRENGTH

1.5 – FRIDAY – LOWER BODY

Welcome to today's **Lower Body Strength** workout! Be sure to drink plenty of water and warm up correctly before starting. Strengthening the leg muscles is vital as you age. Once you begin strengthening these muscles, you may be able to move around with greater ease – improving your overall quality of life! This workout contains several lower-body exercises, such as:

- **Hamstring, groin,** and **quad** muscle exercises
- **Glute, calf,** and **shin** muscle exercises
- **Balance** and **stability** exercises

There are 10 varying exercises with a number of reps to complete for each exercise, so it should take a total of 10 minutes to complete. You can use any chair/table and a small stand or the first step of the stairs for these exercises.

It is advised to use the **Free Audiobook** (once released) as a guide for these workouts, as it is timed and guides you through each exercise.

Please check the video demonstrations using the **QR code on page 29** for correct form and technique. You should never be in pain doing any exercises. Please ensure correct form by stabilizing your core muscles and keeping a bend on your knees and a straight back.

Have a good workout!

1 HAMSTRING KICKS

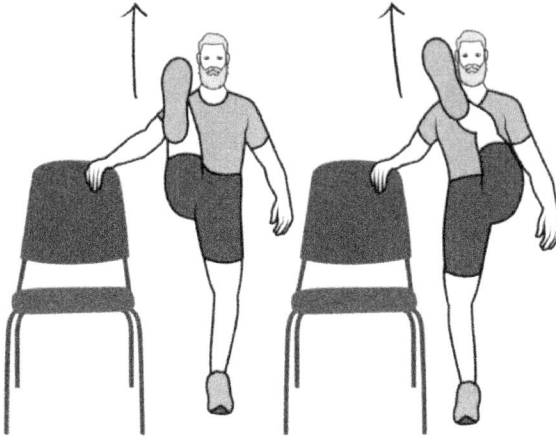

X10 each side

- swinging high kicks

- (hold or wall for balance)

2 STEP UPS

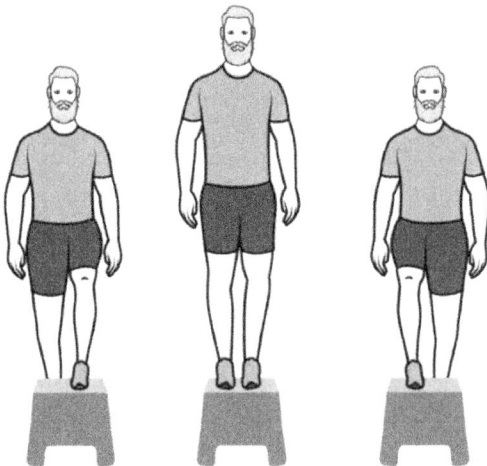

X10 each side

- step ups

- change stepping leg after 10

3 LUNGES

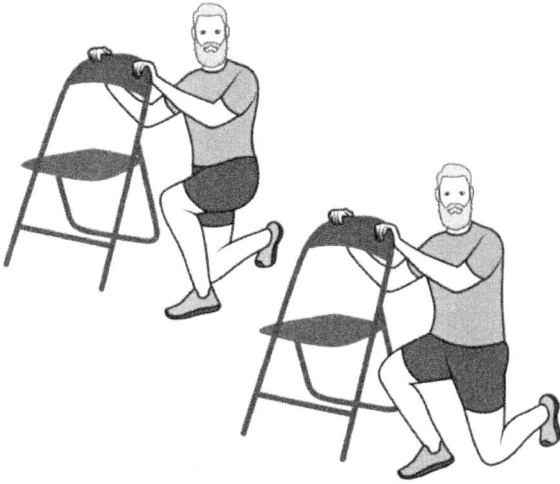

X10 each side

- (use chair or wall for balance)

- Lunge with knee close to or touching ground

4 CALF RAISES (DOUBLE OR SINGLE)

X10 each side

- raise heel(s) off floor + hold for 2 seconds, then drop - (double or single)

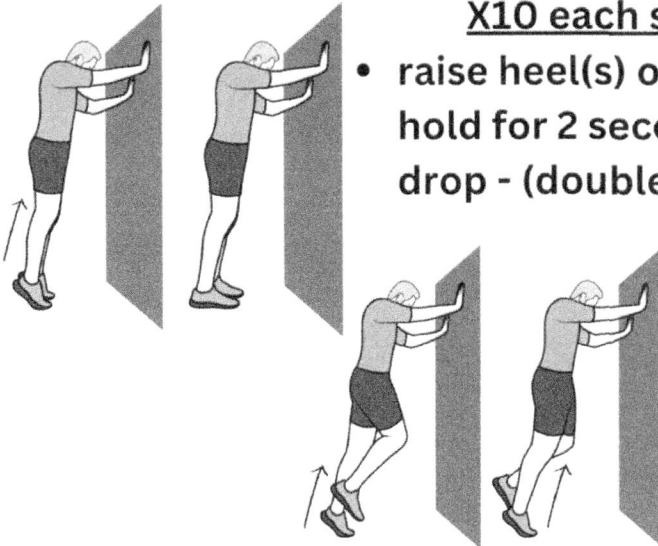

5 SQUATS TO CHAIR

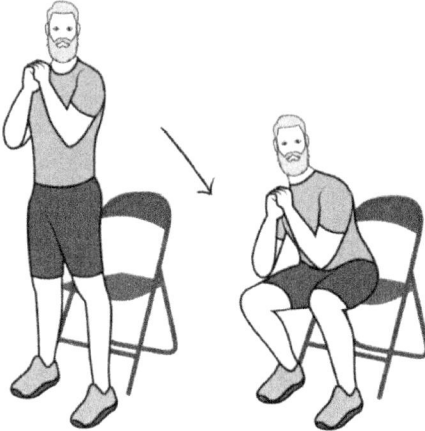

X10

- deep squat to chair
- stand back up

6 BULGARIAN SPLIT SQUAT

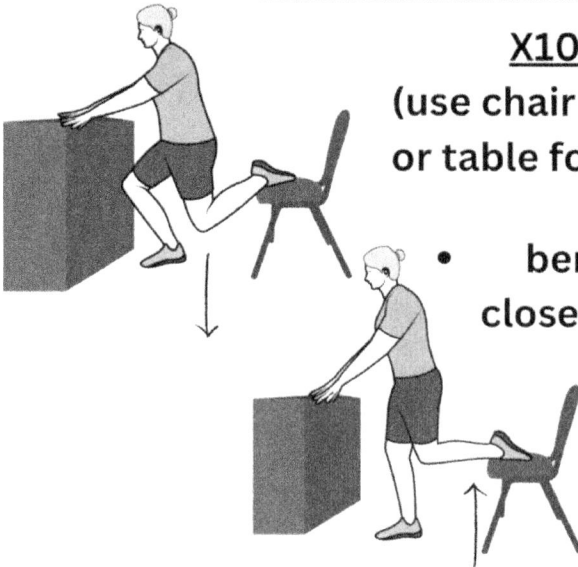

X10 each side
(use chair for foot + wall or table for balance)

- bend knee down close to ground then back up

7

HAMSTRING CURLS

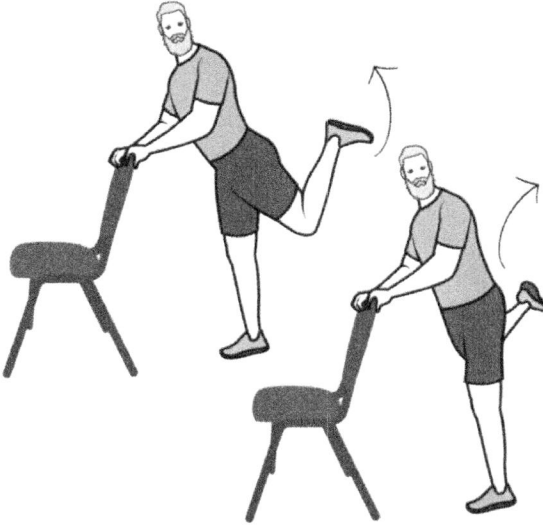

X10 each side

- use chair/wall for balance
- kick back and curl hamstrings left and right

(see video demo)

8

TOE RAISES

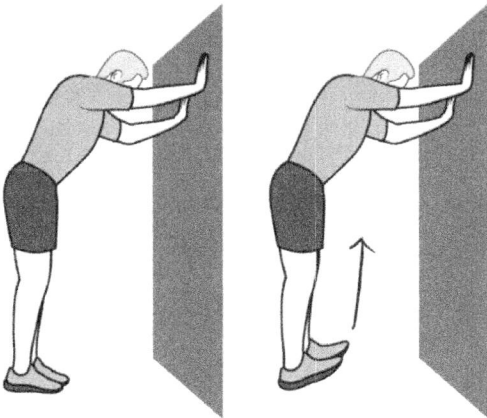

X10

- use wall for balance - point toes to sky and hold for 3 seconds

- (works shin muscles)

9   SIDE LEG RAISES

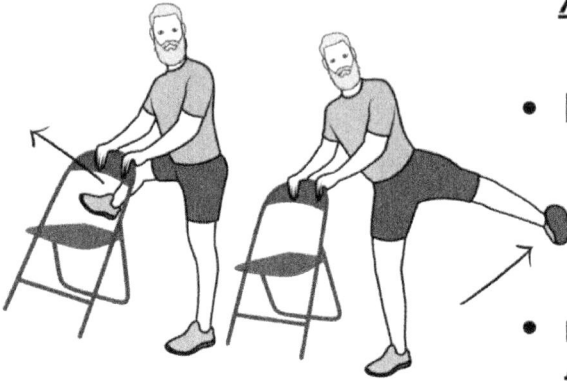

X10 each side

- hold chair/table

- raise foot out to the side and back down

10   GLUTE BRIDGES (DOUBLE OR SINGLE)

DOUBLE

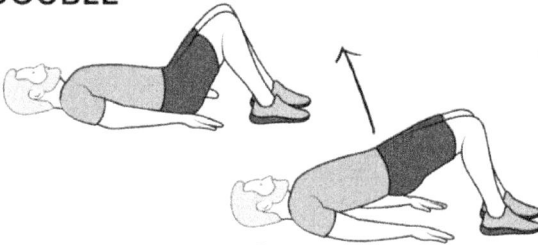

X10

- lie on floor - raise hips to sky + hold for 3 seconds

SINGLE

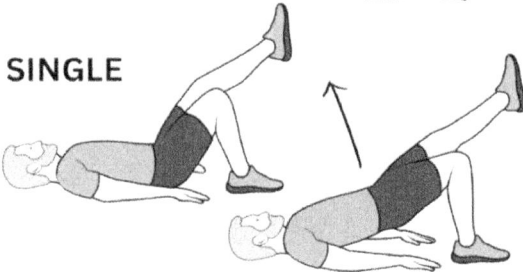

- raise one foot for more difficulty + do each side

1.5 – FRIDAY – LOWER BODY SUMMARY

1 HAMSTRING KICKS

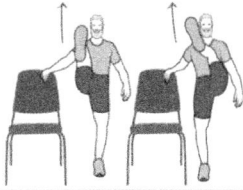

X10 ES

2 STEP-UPS

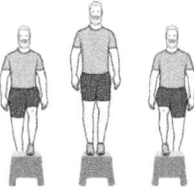

X10 ES

3 LUNGES

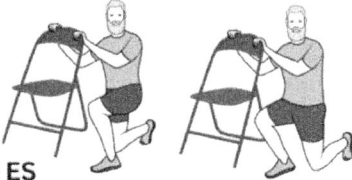

X10 ES

4 CALF RAISES (DOUBLE OR SINGLE)

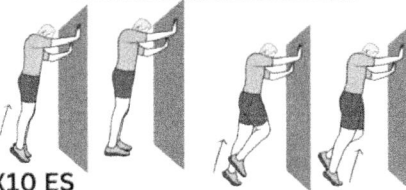

X10 ES

5 SQUATS TO CHAIR

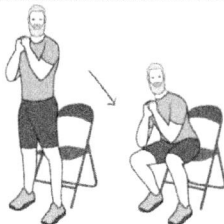

X10

6 BULGARIAN SPLIT SQUAT

X10 ES

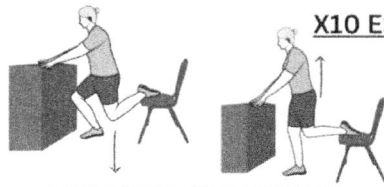

7 HAMSTRING CURLS

X10 ES

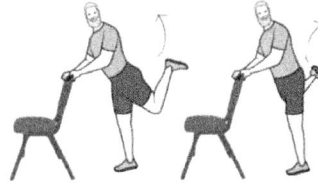

8 TOE RAISES

X10

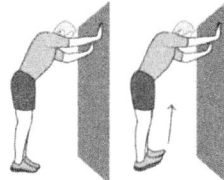

9 SIDE LEG RAISES

X10 ES

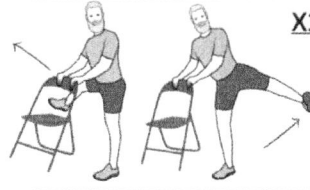

10 GLUTE BRIDGES (DOUBLE OR SINGLE)

DOUBLE
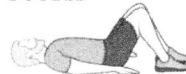
X10
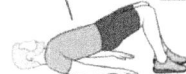

SINGLE
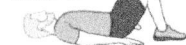
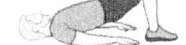

1.6 - SATURDAY - BOXING CARDIO HIIT 2

1.6 – SATURDAY – BOXING HITT 2

Welcome to today's **Boxing Cardio HIIT** session! Today is a fun workout, with every workout inspired by boxing training. It's time to unleash your inner **Rocky**! Today's HIIT workout will include:

- **30 seconds** of high-intensity work
- Followed by **30 seconds** of rest before beginning the next exercise/round.
- **Skipping**, **jogging,** and **head movements** to slip and dodge punches
- Different **punch combinations** to deliver the knockout blow to your enemy!

There are 10 varying exercises (or rounds), so it should take a total of 10 minutes to complete. It is advised to use the **Free Audiobook** (once released) as a guide for these workouts, as it is timed and will tell you when 30 seconds are up for each round.

If you are doing this workout for the first time, it is ok to go at a **medium intensity** for the first few rounds. Slowly over time, you can increase the intensity. You want to push yourself just outside your comfort zone each round. Each week you will notice an improvement.

Please check the video demonstrations using the **QR code on page 29** for the correct form and technique of each exercise.

Have a good workout!

1 **RUNING ON THE SPOT**

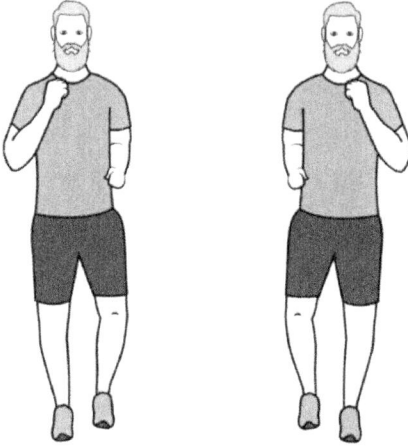

<u>30s on/30s off</u>

- running on the spot

2 **JUMPING JACKS**

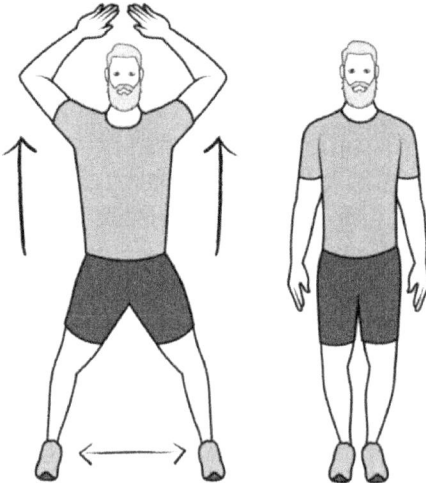

<u>30s on/30s off</u>

- jumping jacks continuously

3 SKIPPING

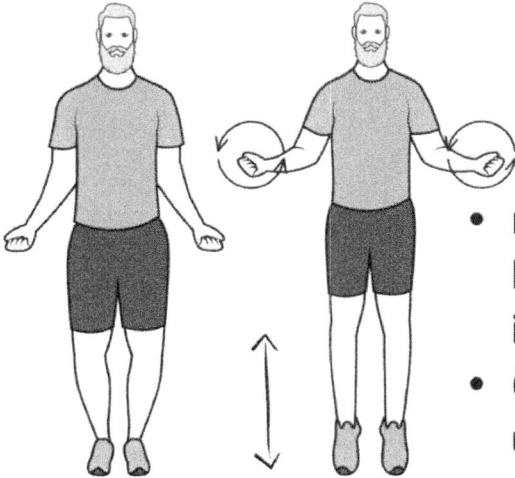

30s on/30s off

- replicate skipping by jumping over an imaginary rope
- (twist wrists + jump up and down)

4 CROSS PUNCHES

30s on/30s off

- left hand cross punch + left foot step out
- change to right hand/right foot - repeat

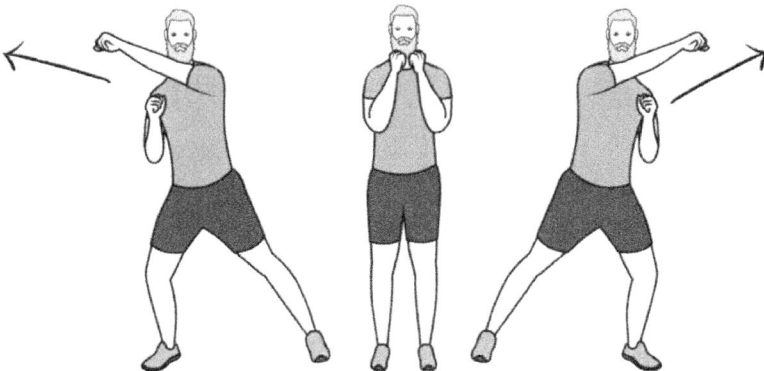

5   SIDE STEP HOOK

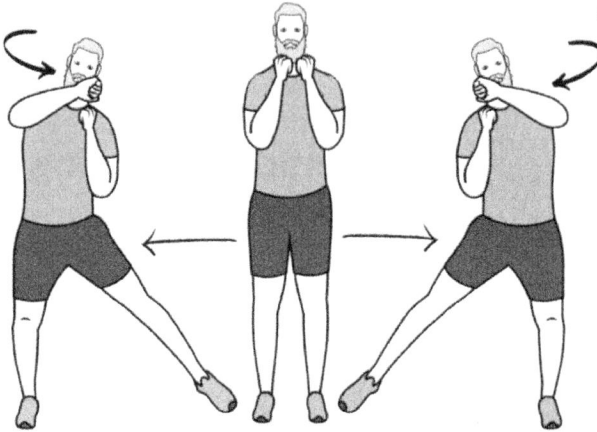

30s on/30s off

- step right -
  hook right
  hand -
  change step
  left hook left
  hand

(see video
demo)

6   TRICEP FLYS

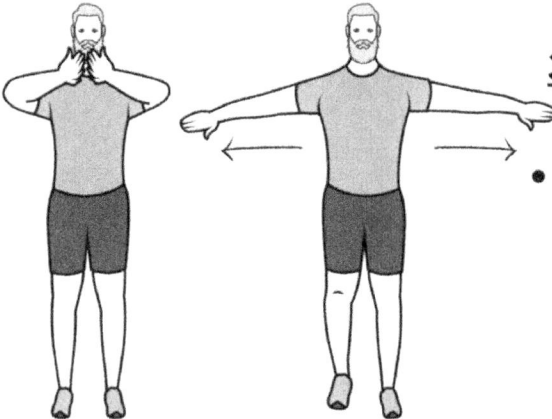

30s on/30s off

- press arms out
  straight to
  sides with
  triceps
  continuously

7 DUCK AND WEAVE

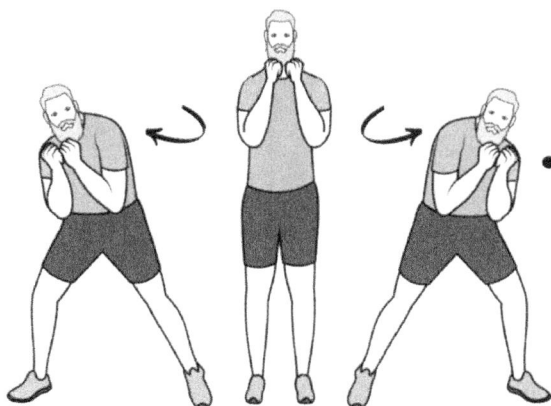

30s on/30s off

- boxers stance - duck right and left with hands up protecting

(see video demo)

8 UPPERCUTS

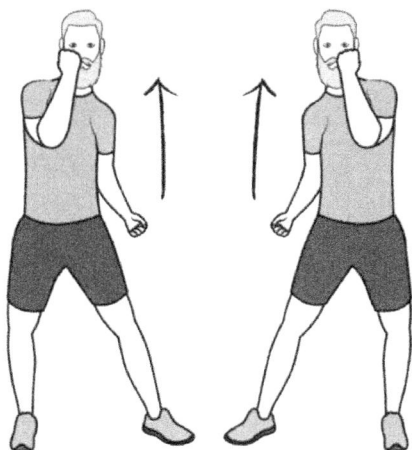

30s on/30s off

- continuous uppercuts right + left

(see video demo)

9

4 PUNCH COMBO - JAB-JAB-HOOK-HOOK

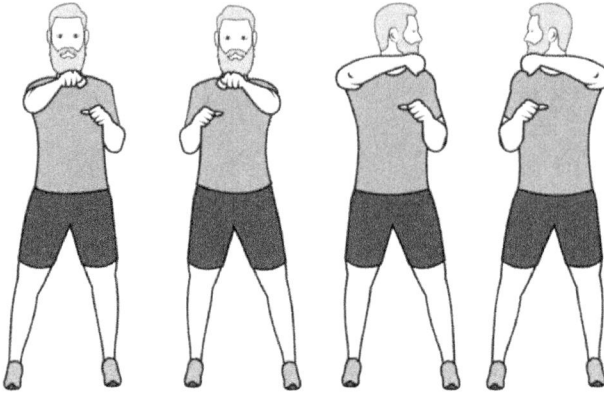

- right jab/
- left jab/
- right hook/
- left hook

30s on/30s off

repeat

10

RUNNING ON THE SPOT

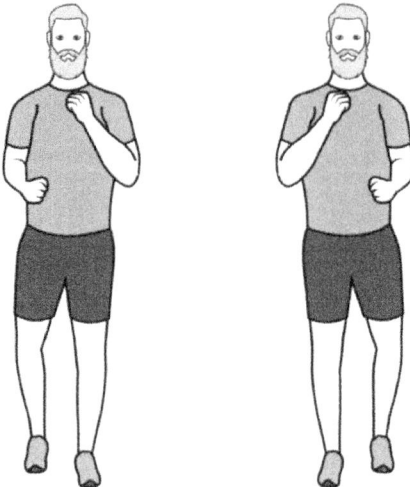

30s on/30s off

- running on the spot
- finish with a fast pace

1.6 – SATURDAY – BOXING HIIT 2 SUMMARY

1 RUNNING ON THE SPOT

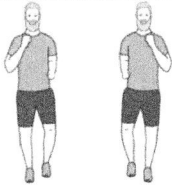

30 SEC WORK

6 TRICEP FLYS

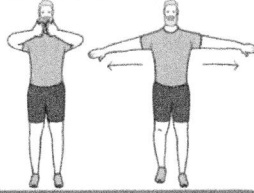

30 SEC REST

2 JUMPING JACKS

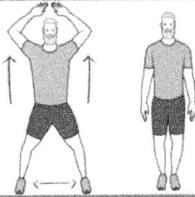

7 DUCK AND WEAVE

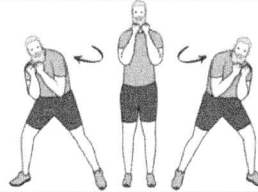

3 SKIPPING

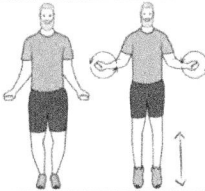

8 UPPERCUTS

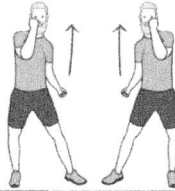

4 CROSS PUNCHES

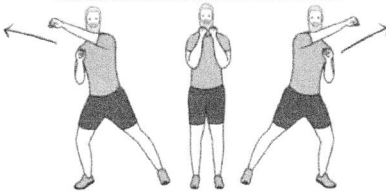

9 4 PUNCH COMBO JAB-JAB-HOOK-HOOK

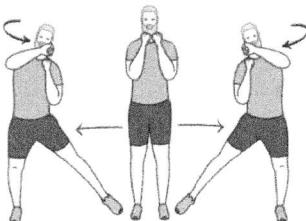

5 SIDE STEP- HOOK

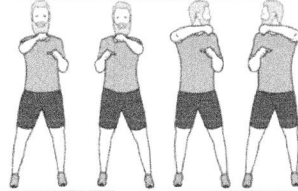

10 RUNNING ON THE SPOT

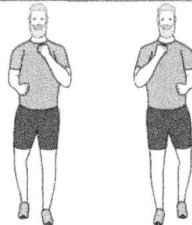

BRIAN HARDY

1.7 - SUNDAY - YOGA

1.7 – SUNDAY - YOGA

Welcome to today's **Yoga** session! Sunday is a day to relax and rejuvenate the mind and body, and this yoga session will help you to do just that. Be sure to drink water and warm up correctly before starting. Yoga is an amazing way to control your breathing, ease your mind, and help the body become used to moving into different positions. Today's yoga session will consist of the following:

- **Slow and controlled** stretches and movements
- **Engaging your core** muscles
- **Controlled breathing** with slow **inhales and exhales**
- **Loosening of the hips, spine,** and much more

There are 10 varying yoga poses, so it should take approximately 10 minutes to complete. This workout is all about calming the mind and body. Follow the steps provided. Some exercises will contain timed holds, while others will have repetitions.

It is advised to use the **Free Audiobook** (once released) as a guide for these workouts, as it is timed and guides you through each exercise.

Please check the video demonstrations using the **QR code on page 29**, for correct form and technique.

Namaste!

1 SIDE REACHES

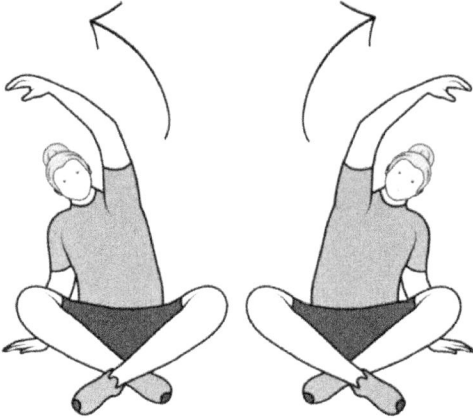

X2 each side

- use other hand for balance - reach over head + hold for 5 seconds each time

2 NECK STRETCHES

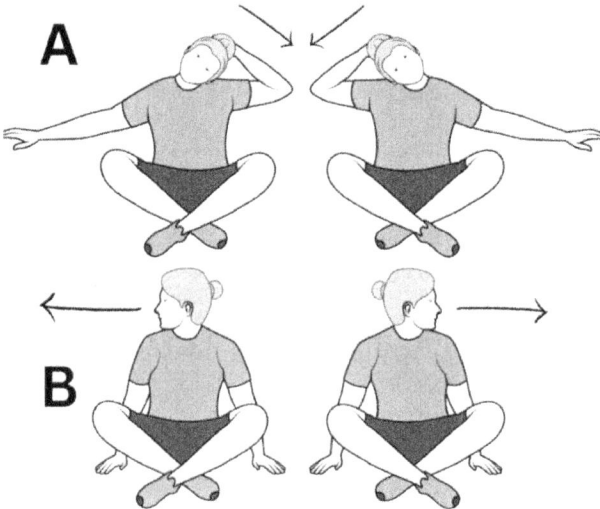

A

B

X2 each side
<u>A</u> - tilt head + light pull down + hold for 5 seconds

<u>B</u> - look to the side + hold for 5 seconds

3 CAT/CAMEL

X5 each
- **slow + controlled cat camel poses for 5-10 seconds time**

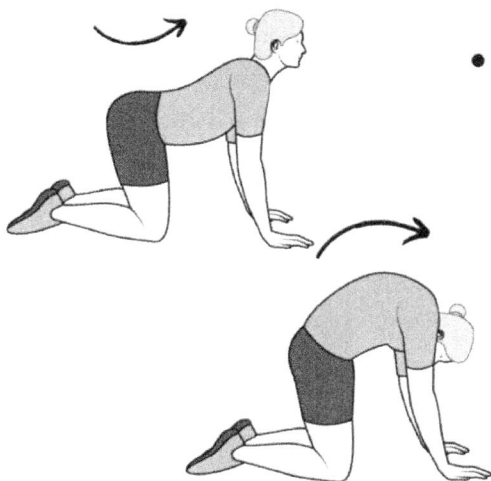

4 CHILDS POSE

30+ seconds
- **reach hands forward + sit back into childs pose for 30+ seconds**

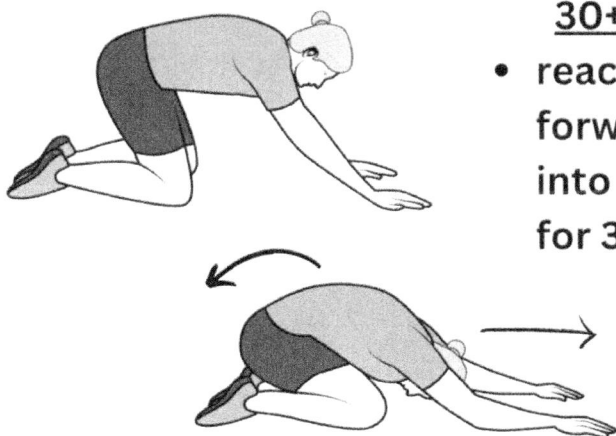

5 TOE REACH LOOSEN

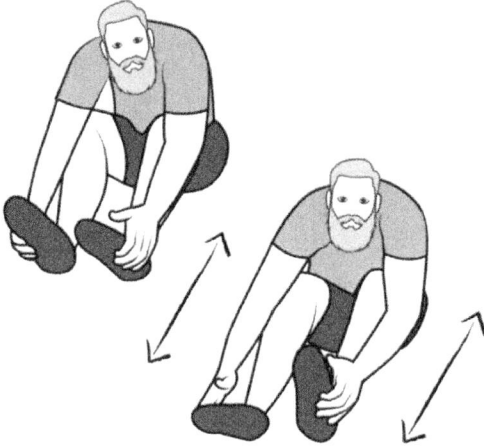

30+ seconds

- bend knees and grab feet - walk out feet for 30+ seconds

6 HALF LORD TWIST

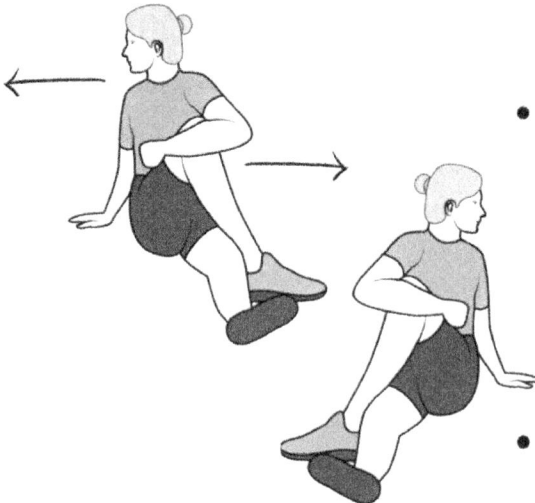

X2 each side

- right leg over left - twist body right as far as possible + hold for 30 seconds

- change to opposite side

7 KNEE HUG AND ROCK

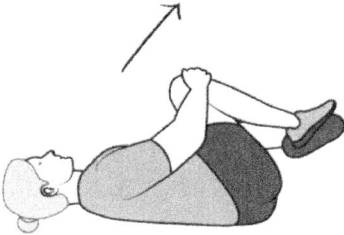

30 seconds

- lie back - hug knees to chest + rock side to side for 30+ seconds

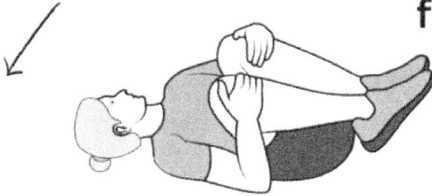

8 GLUTE BRIDGE

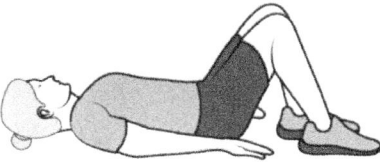

30 seconds

- raise hips to sky for glute bridge + hold for 20-30 seconds

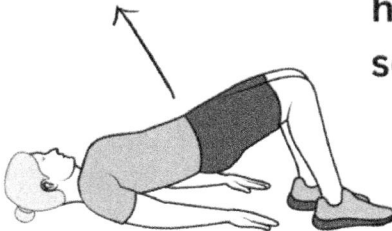

9 HAPPY BABY

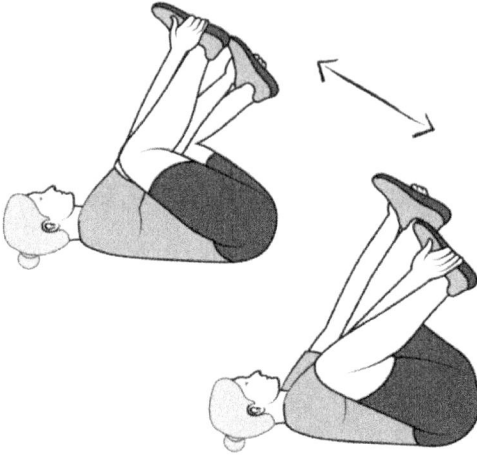

30+ seconds
- bend knees, grab feet + walk out and rock for 30-50 seconds

10 FULL BODY STRETCH

30+ seconds
- lie down flat then stretch arms + legs out for 20 - 30 seconds

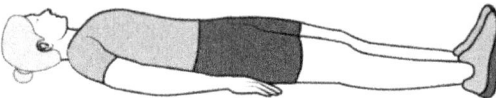

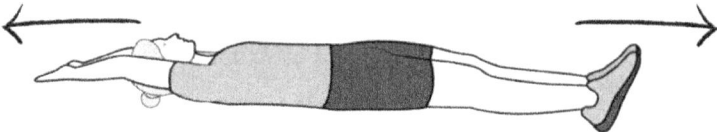

Namaste!

1.7 – SUNDAY – YOGA SUMMARY

1 SIDE REACHES

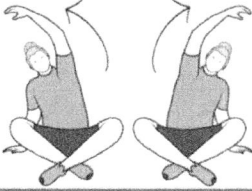

X2 ES
5 SEC

2 NECK STRETCHES

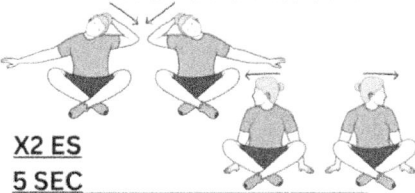

X2 ES
5 SEC

3 CAT/CAMEL

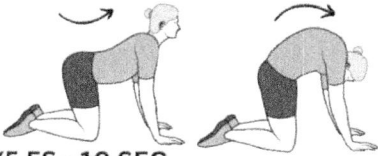

X5 ES - 10 SEC

4 CHILDS POSE

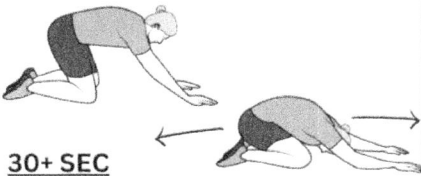

30+ SEC

5 TOE REACH LOOSEN

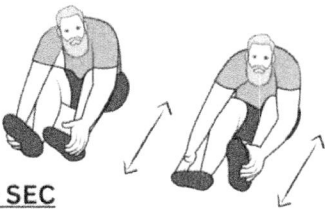

30+ SEC

6 HALF LORD TWIST

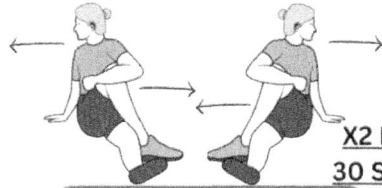

X2 ES
30 SEC

7 KNEE HUG AND ROCK

30+ SEC

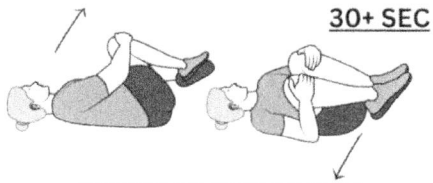

8 GLUTE BRIDGE

30 SEC

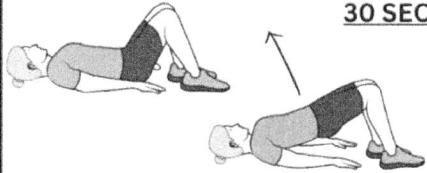

9 HAPPY BABY

30+ SEC

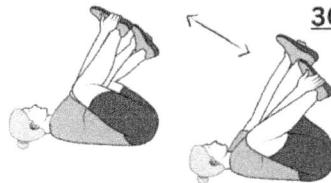

10 FULL BODY STRETCH

30+ SEC

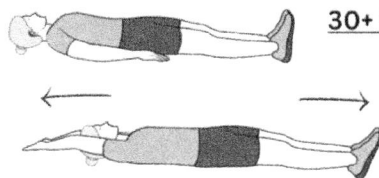

Namaste!

BRIAN HARDY

INTERLUDE

At this point in the book, I have a small favor to ask. As there are many similar books in this category, I have learned that gathering reviews is hugely important.

If you like what you have read so far, and it has brought some value and knowledge to your life, it would be extremely helpful and valuable if you could take 30 seconds of your time and head over to Amazon and write a nice brief review. A sentence or two will do!

This way, it can reach more people and help them lead a healthier lifestyle.

Just scan the QR code with your phone camera and it will take you straight to the review section.

Thank you! You have my heartfelt gratitude. I look forward to seeing your thoughts.

BRIAN HARDY

LEVEL 2

2.0 - STANDARD WARM-UP

2.0 – STANDARD WARM-UP

Welcome to your standard warm-up! This warm-up contains 10 simple stretches and exercises to warm up your muscles and get the blood flowing. By doing the given routine, your joints will be loosened up, and you will be ready to work out and push your body outside its comfort zone. It's essential you do this full standard warm-up before every workout. This warm-up contains the following:

- Loosening your **shoulders**, **spine,** and other joint areas
- **Stretching** your upper body and lower body muscles
- **Loosening** out any stiff areas
- And more…

It is advised to use the **Free Audiobook** (once released) as a guide for these workouts, as it is timed and guides you through each exercise.

Please check the video demonstrations using the **QR code on page 29** for the correct form and technique. After some time, these exercises will become second nature, and you will instantly know what to do.

Have a good warm-up!

1 SHAKE IT OUT

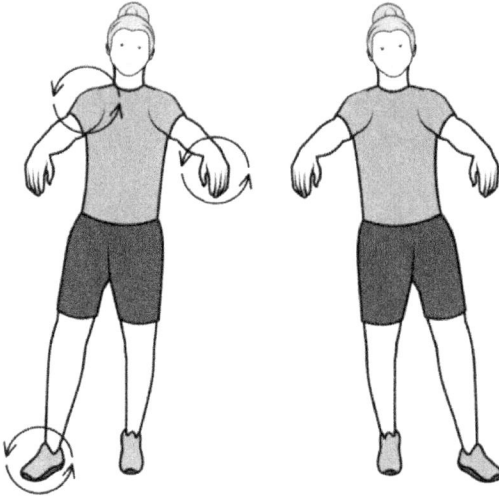

15+ Seconds

- shake / loosen arms + legs

2 SHOULDER ROTATIONS

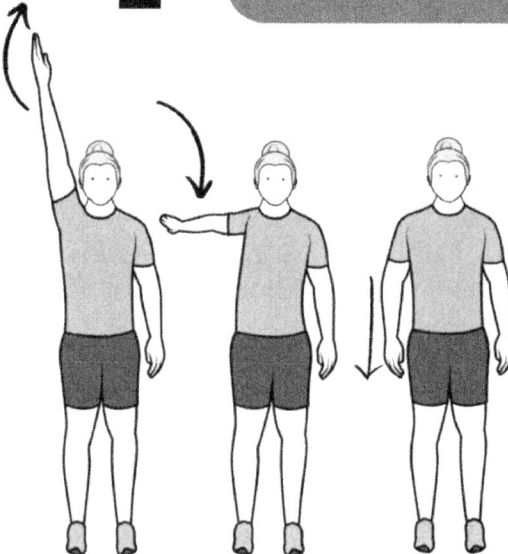

X3 each side

- full rotations around and back around on each arm

- (see video demo)

3 CROSS ARM STRETCH

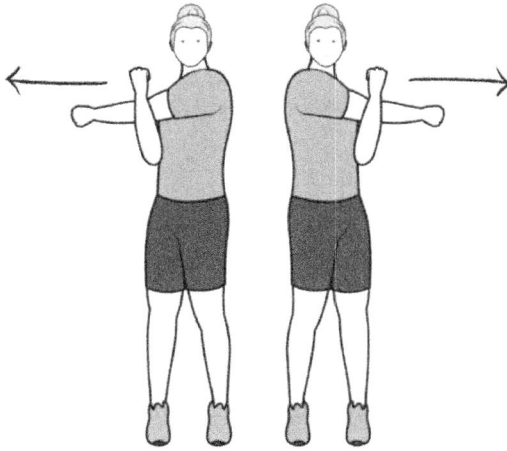

X2 each side

- cross arm across chest
- 5-second holds each side

4 HAMSTRING STRETCH

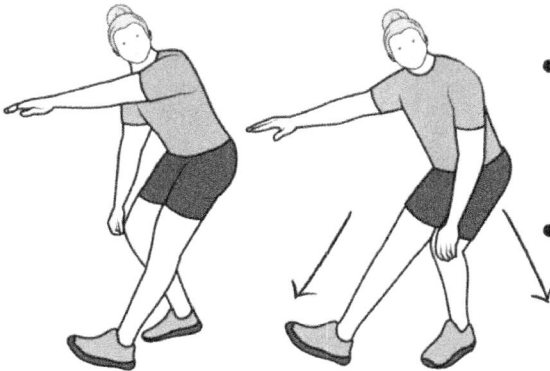

X3 each side

- 5-second holds on each leg
- Sit back - lock out leg - toe facing up - hand out

5 GROIN STRETCH

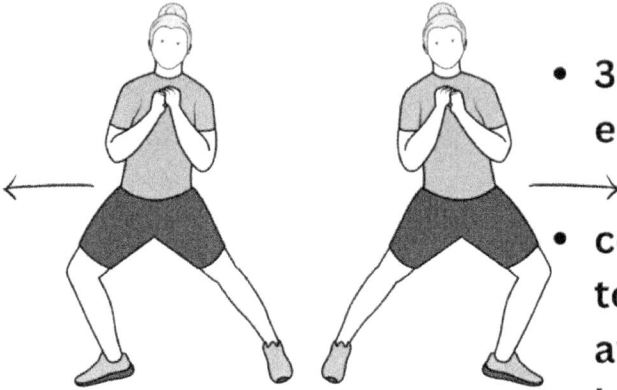

X3 each side

- 3-second holds each side

- core engaged, toe pointing away on bent leg

6 CALF STRETCH

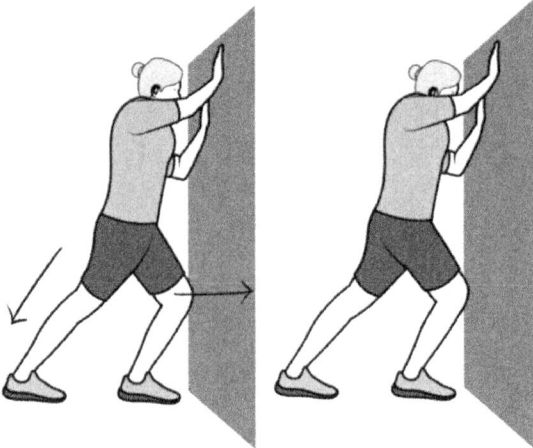

X2 each side

- 10-second hold each leg

- push knee to wall + lock out knee on back leg + heel to ground

7 CHEST ROTATIONS

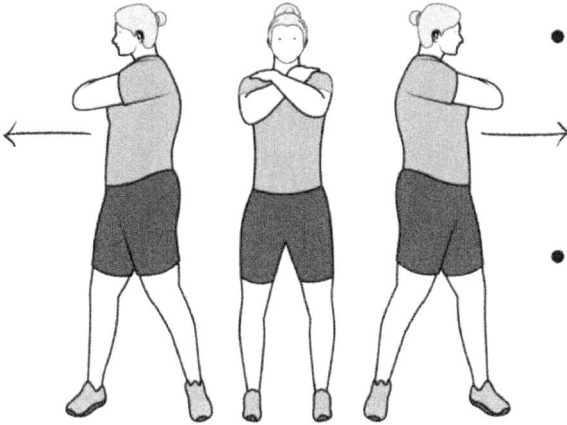

<u>X3 each side</u>

- cross arms + rotate upper body

- (5 second hold on each twist - back straight + core engaged)

8 REACH UP -> TOE TOUCH

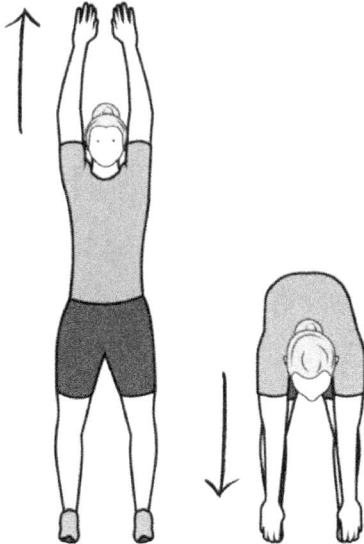

<u>X2</u>

- reach tall as possible on tippy toes

  +

- fold down slowly and touch your shin/toes

9 RUNNING ON THE SPOT

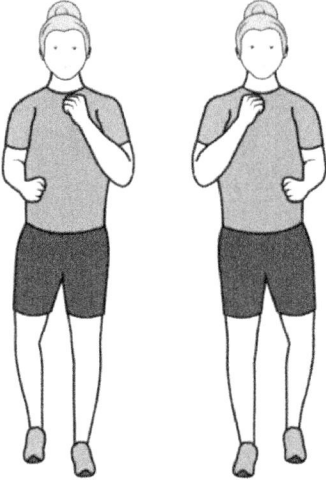

15+ seconds

- jogging on the spot

10 SHAKE IT OUT

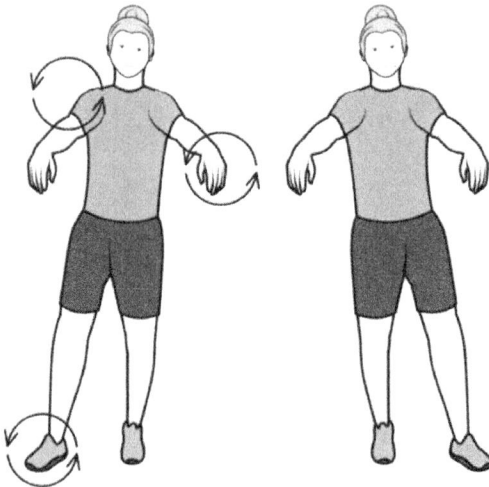

15+ Seconds

- shake / loosen arms + legs

2.0 – WARM-UP SUMMARY

1 SHAKE IT OUT

15+ SEC

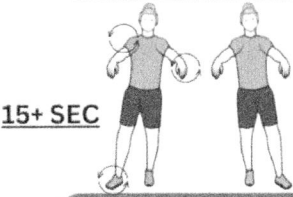

2 SHOULDER ROTATIONS

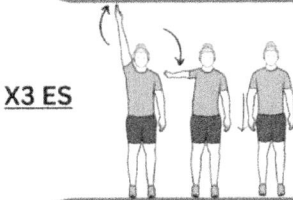

X3 ES

3 CROSS ARM STRETCH

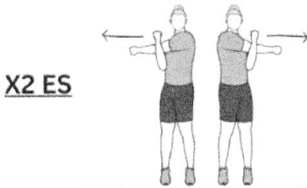

X2 ES

4 HAMSTRING STRETCH

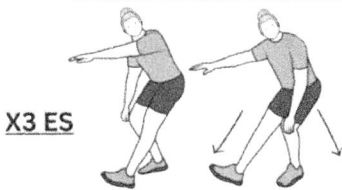

X3 ES

5 GROIN STRETCH

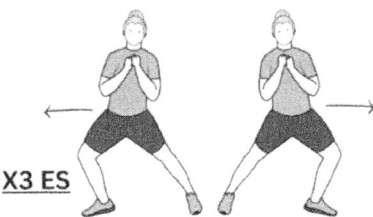

X3 ES

6 CALF STRETCH

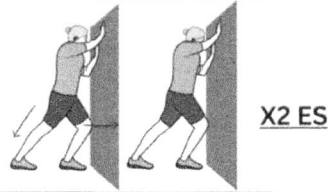

X2 ES

7 CHEST ROTATIONS

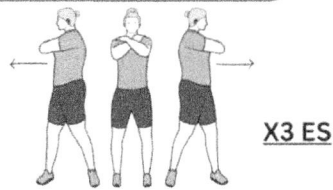

X3 ES

8 REACH UP -> TOE TOUCH

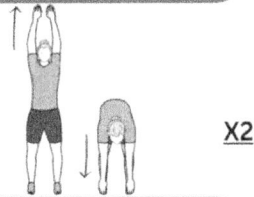

X2

9 RUNNING ON THE SPOT

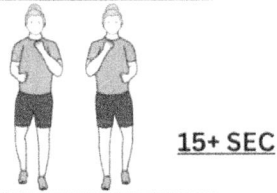

15+ SEC

10 SHAKE IT OUT

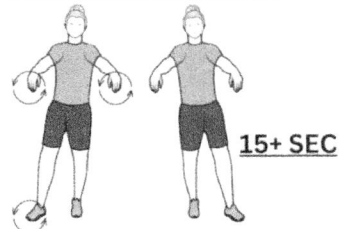

15+ SEC

BRIAN HARDY

2.1 - MONDAY - UPPER BODY STRENGTH

2.1 – MONDAY – UPPER BODY

Welcome to **Monday's Upper Body Strength** Day! Be sure to drink plenty of water and warm up correctly before starting. This workout contains several upper-body exercises such as:

- **Bicep, tricep,** and **shoulder** exercises
- **Back** and **chest** exercises
- **Stability** exercises using your **core muscles** for correct form and technique

There are 10 varying exercises with a number of reps to complete for each exercise, so it should take a total of 10 minutes to complete. All you need is 2 cans of food, 2 water bottles, or anything that weighs a few KG – That's it!

It is advised to use the **Free Audiobook** (once released) as a guide for these workouts, as it is timed and guides you through each exercise.

Please check the video demonstrations using the **QR code on page 29** for correct form and technique. You should never be in pain doing any exercises. Please ensure correct form by stabilizing your core muscles and keeping a bend on your knees and a straight back.

Have a good workout!

1 **WALL PUSH-UPS**

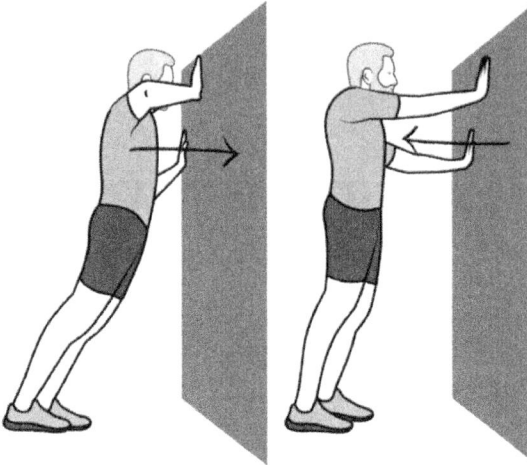

X14

- lean chest close to wall

- push out + lock elbows

2 **SHOULDER BLADE SQUEEZES**

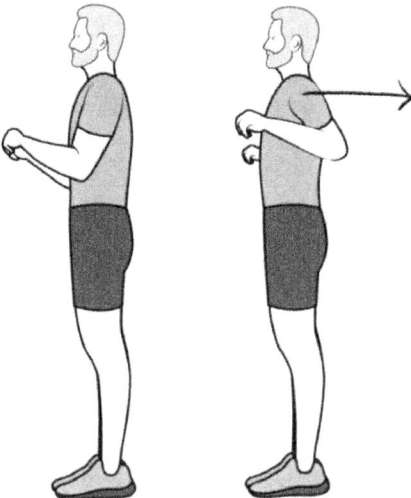

X14
(focus on shoulder blades)

- pull elbows back + squeeze shoulder blades for 3 seconds

3 BICEP CURLS

<u>X14</u>

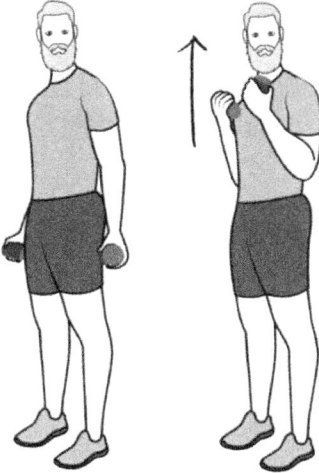

- bend elbows + curl biceps up and down

(use cans of food or bottles of water or light dumbbells)

4 BENT OVER ROWS

<u>X14</u>

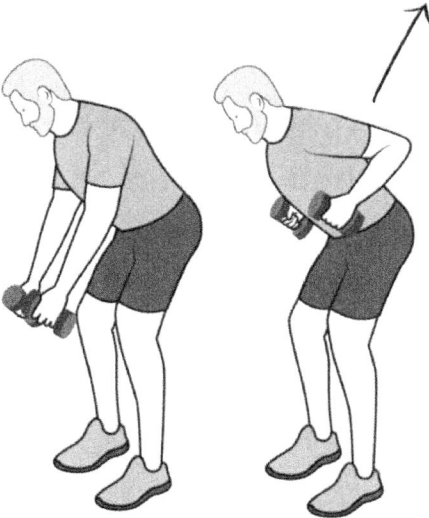

- slight lean forward + bend knees + engage core + straight back

- squeeze shoulder blades + 10 rows with cans/bottles /weights

5   CHEST PRESS

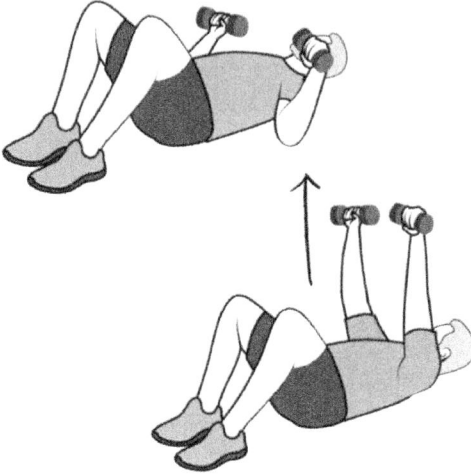

X14

- lie down on floor + bend knees

- bend elbows to touch floor then press up straight and down

6   TRICEP EXTENSIONS

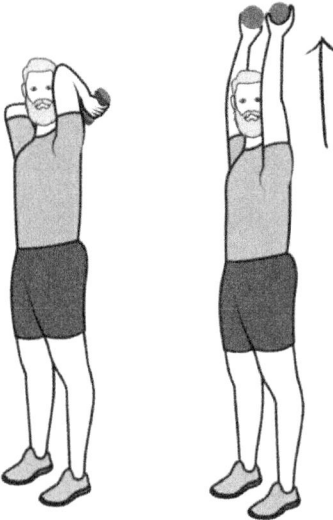

X14

- hold cans/bottles behind head as shown, bend elbows then extend up using triceps

- (engage core + straight back)

7 SHOULDER PRESS

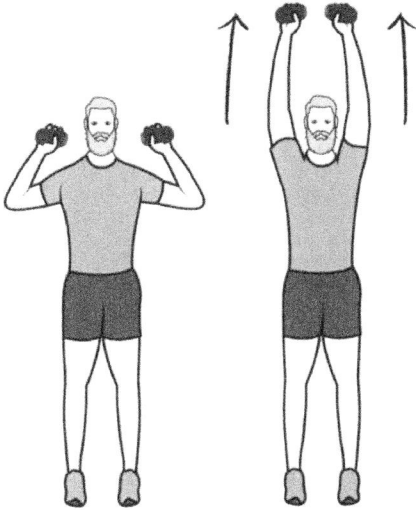

X14

- hold cans/bottles to side of head as shown + extend overhead locking arms up

- (engage core + straight back)

8 CHEST FLYS

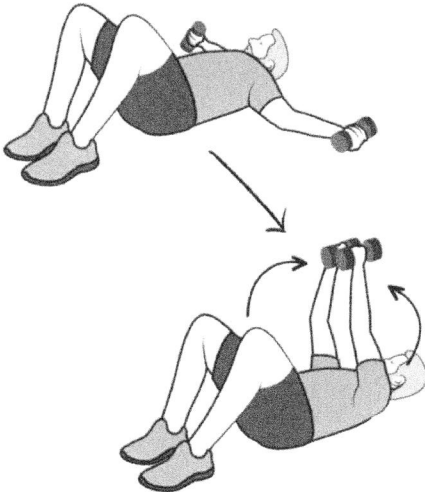

X14

- (lie down on floor + bend knees)

- hold cans straight out touching the ground as shown

- press cans together keeping arms straight

9 REVERSE FLYS

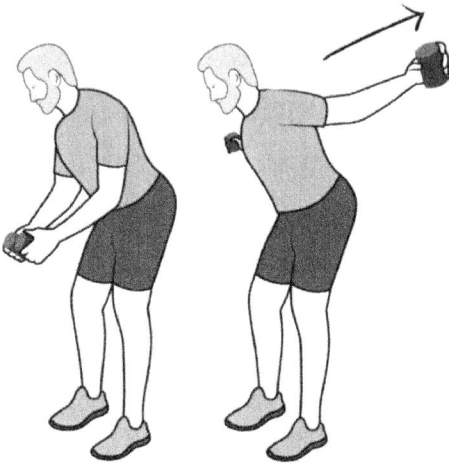

X14
- slight lean forward + bend knees + engage core + straight back
- squeeze shoulder blades + fly back cans as shown + keep arms straight

10 SHOULDER RAISES

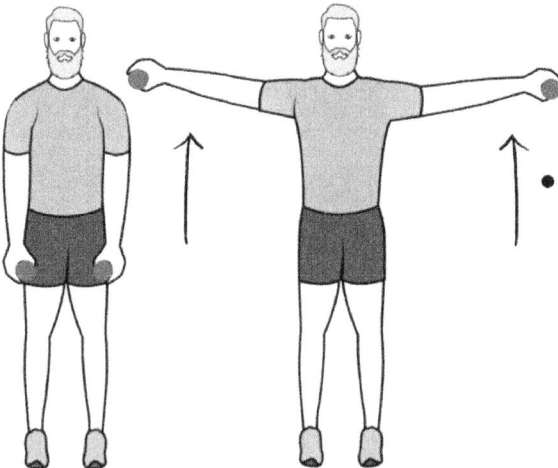

X14
- raise cans up and down with arms straight out to the side using shoulder strength

2.1 – MONDAY – UPPER BODY SUMMARY

1 WALL PUSH-UPS

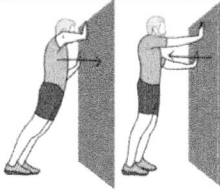

X14

6 TRICEP EXTENSIONS

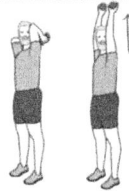

X14

2 SHOULDER BLADE SQUEEZES

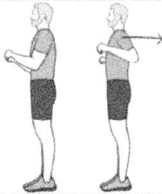

X14

7 SHOULDER PRESS

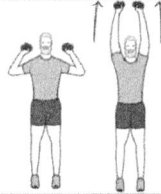

X14

3 BICEP CURLS

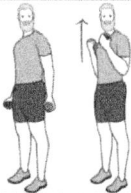

X14

8 CHEST FLYS

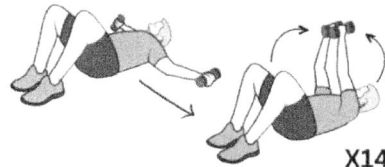

X14

4 BENT OVER ROWS

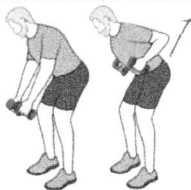

X14

9 REVERSE FLYS

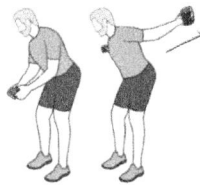

X14

5 CHEST PRESS

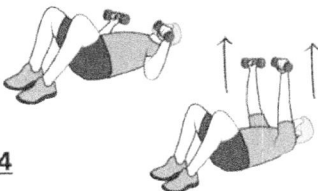

X14

10 SHOULDER RAISES

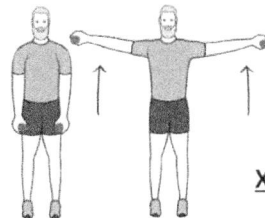

X14

2.2 - TUESDAY - CARDIO HIIT 1

2.2 – TUESDAY – CARDIO HIIT 1

Welcome to **Tuesday's Cardio HIIT** session number 1 of the week! Be sure to drink plenty of water and warm up correctly before starting. This workout will be timed at intervals. As a High-Intensity Interval Training session, this workout will follow this path:

- **35 seconds** of high-intensity work
- Followed by **25 seconds** of rest before beginning the next exercise/round.

There are 10 varying exercises (or rounds), so it should take a total of 10 minutes to complete. You can use a small stand or the first step of the stairs for the step-ups exercises

It is advised to use the **Free Audiobook** (once released) as a guide for these workouts, as it is timed and will tell you when 30 seconds are up for each round. The timer on phones can be awkward as the screen locks, and you cannot see the time.

If you are doing this workout for the first time, it is ok to go at a **medium intensity** for the first few rounds. Slowly over time, you can increase the intensity. You want to push yourself just outside your comfort zone each round. Each week you will notice an improvement.

Please check the video demonstrations using the **QR code on page 29** for the correct form and technique of each exercise. Have a good workout!

1 RUNNING ON THE SPOT

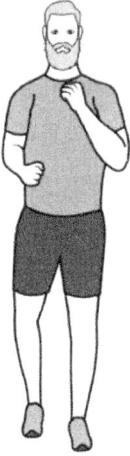 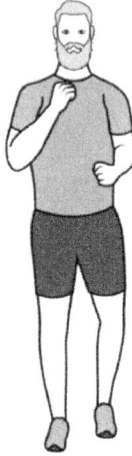

35s on/25s off

- running on the spot

2 STEP UPS

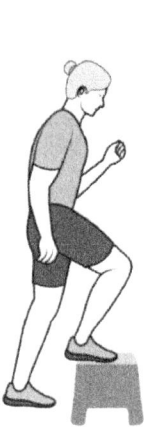 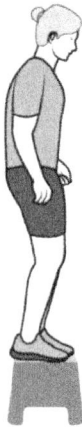 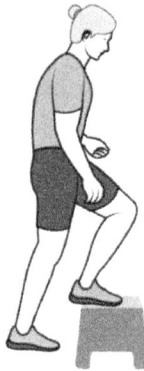

35s on/25s off

- use box + step up and down quick

- (change stepping foot every 5 steps)

3

**CRUNCHES
KNEE TO ELBOW**

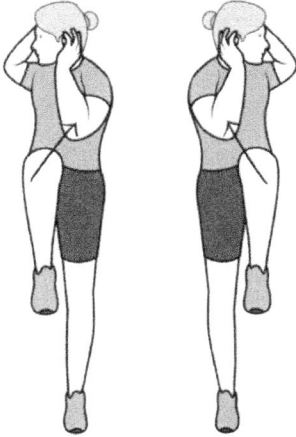

35s on/25s off

- hands to side of head - try touch elbow to opposite knee

- alternate each side

4

PUNCH UP -> PUNCH OUT

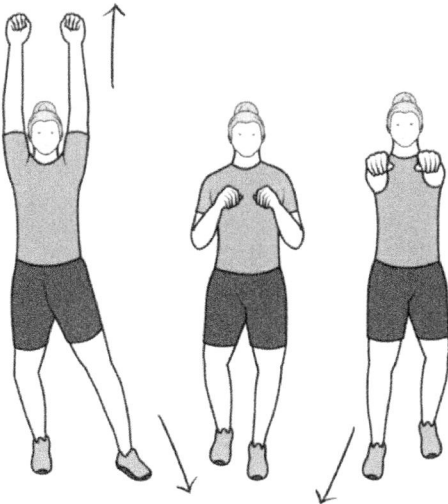

35s on/25s off

- punch up + toe tap to one side

- punch out + toe tap to other side

5 SQUATS

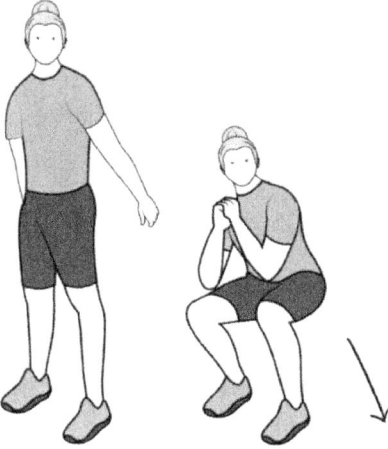

35s on/25s off

- squat as low as possible then straight back up

- (use a chair to squat on if you need)

6 SIDE STEPS

35s on/25s off

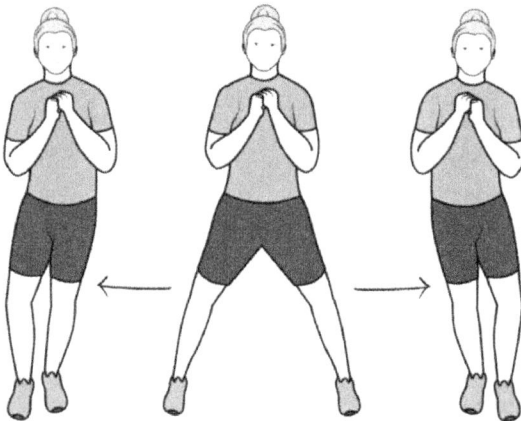

- continuously stepping from side to side

- (see video demo)

7 — LEG CURL AND PRESS

35s on/25s off

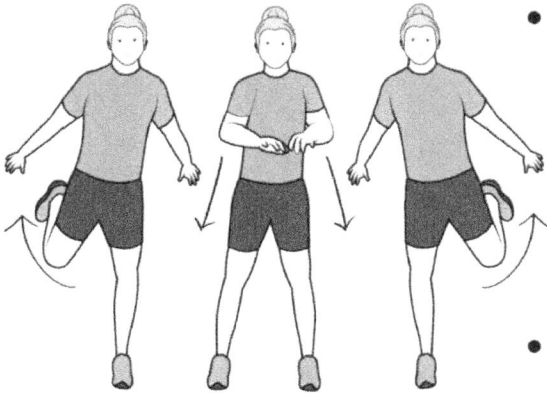

- press elbows up and down with triceps + hamstring curls left and right

- (see video demo)

8 — PUSH FORWARD AND OUT

35s on/25s off

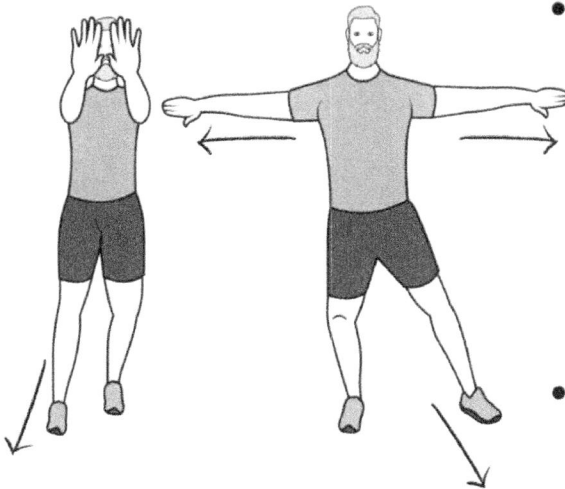

- push forward + step one side then push out to the side + step to other side -

- (see video demo)

9 JUMPING JACKS

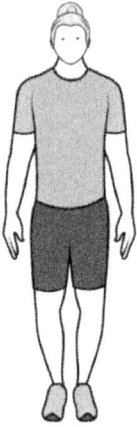

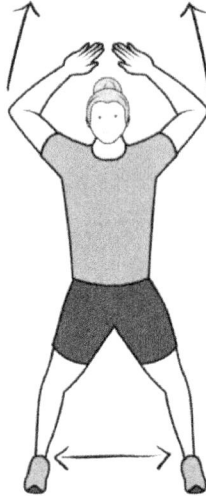

35s on/25s off

- legs out + hands over head

- continuous

10 RUNNING ON THE SPOT

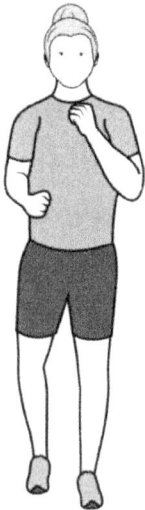

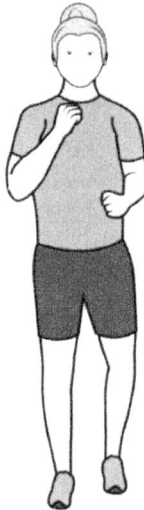

35s on/25s off

- running on the spot at fast pace to finish

2.2 – TUESDAY – CARDIO HIIT 1 SUMMARY

1 RUNNING ON THE SPOT

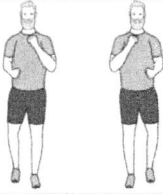

35 SEC WORK   **25 SEC REST**

6 SIDE STEPS

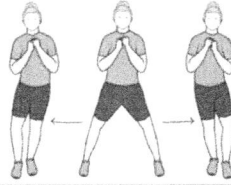

2 STEP-UPS

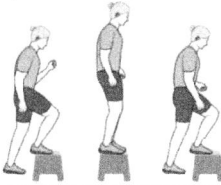

7 LEG CURL AND PRESS

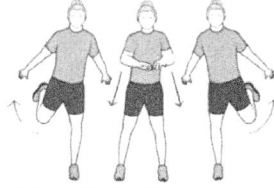

3 CRUNCHES KNEE TO ELBOW

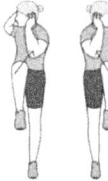

8 PUSH FORWARD AND OUT

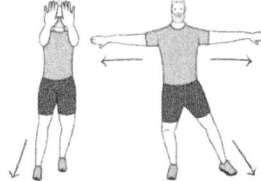

4 PUNCH UP-> PUNCH OUT

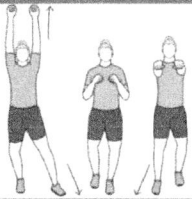

9 JUMPING JACKS

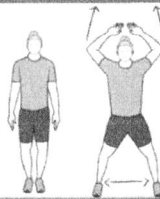

5 SQUATS

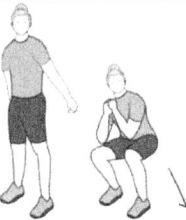

10 RUNNING ON THE SPOT

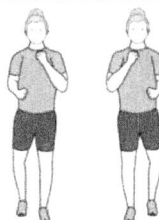

2.3 - WEDNESDAY - BACK RELEASE STRETCHES

2.3 – WEDNESDAY – BACK RELEASE

Welcome to today's **Back Release Stretching** session! Be sure to drink water and warm up correctly before starting. Having a healthy back and spine is crucial to your quality of life. It's all about getting fluid back into your spine and other joints through movement. Today's stretching session will contain the following:

- **Slow and controlled** movements of the joints and spine
- **Engaging your core**
- **Holding deep stretches** in certain positions to release any tension
- And more…

There are 10 **varying** exercises, so it should take approximately 10 minutes to complete. This will be a less intense workout, but keeping a good posture and engaging your core muscles is still crucial. Follow the steps provided. Some exercises will contain timed holds, while others will have repetitions.

It is advised to use the **Free Audiobook** (once released) as a guide for these workouts, as it is timed and guides you through each exercise.

Please check the video demonstrations using the **QR code on page 29** for the correct form and technique of each exercise.

Have a good workout!

1 SHOULDER BLADE ELBOW ROTATIONS

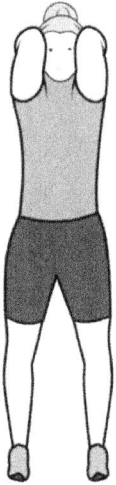

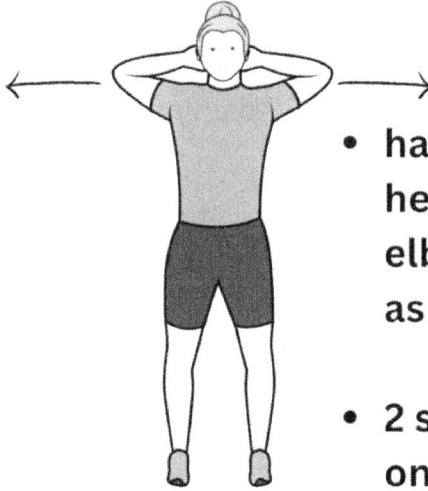

X10

- hands behind head - rotate elbows in and out as shown

- 2 second holds on each rotation

2 HANDS BEHIND HEAD- SIDE TO SIDE

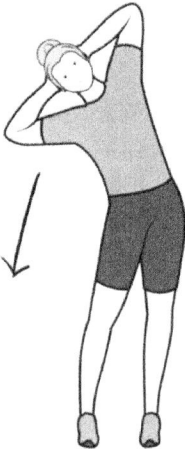

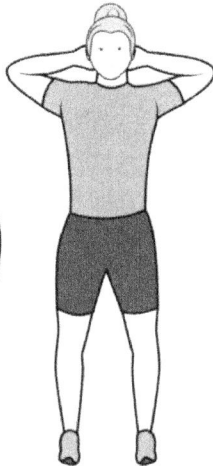

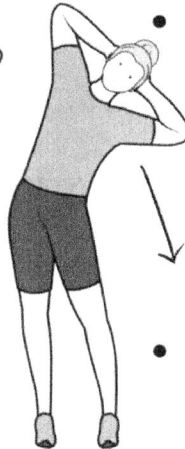

X5 each side

- hands behind head - slowly bend down to side and hold for 3 seconds

- (engage core + straight back)

3 CAT/CAMEL STANDING

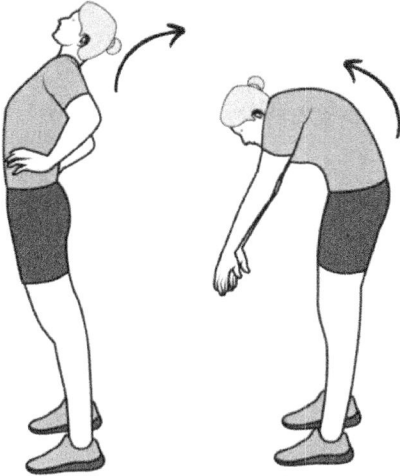

<u>X10</u>
- hand on back, look up + arch back
- change to reach down + round back
- (slow movements)

4 OBLIQUE TWIST AND HOLD

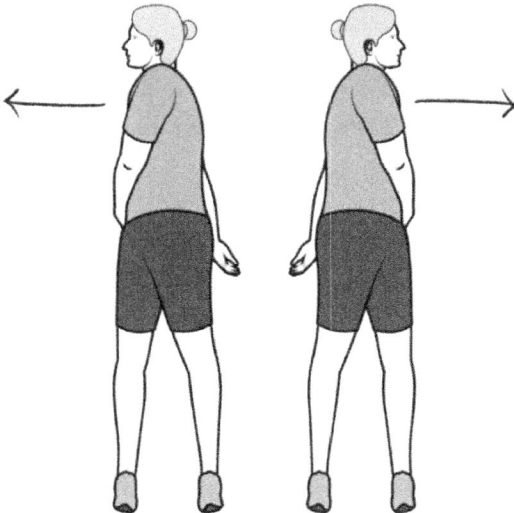

<u>X5 each side</u>
- twist upper body to one side and hold for 5 seconds

5 TALL TO BEND OVER

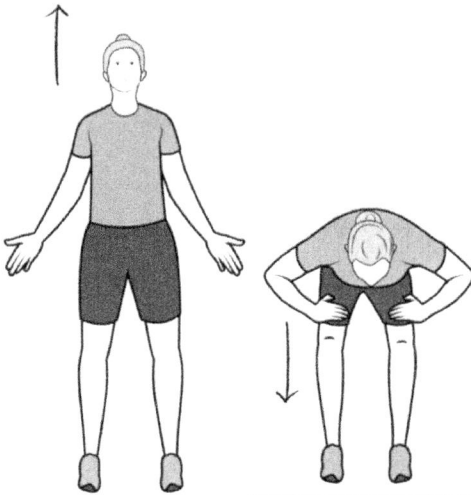

<u>X10</u>
- on tippy toes, stand up tall looking up for 5 seconds

- slowly bend down, hands on legs and hold for 5 seconds

6 SWIMMER REACHES

<u>X10 each side</u>
- wide stance - reach one hand to one side and hold for 2 seconds - change sides

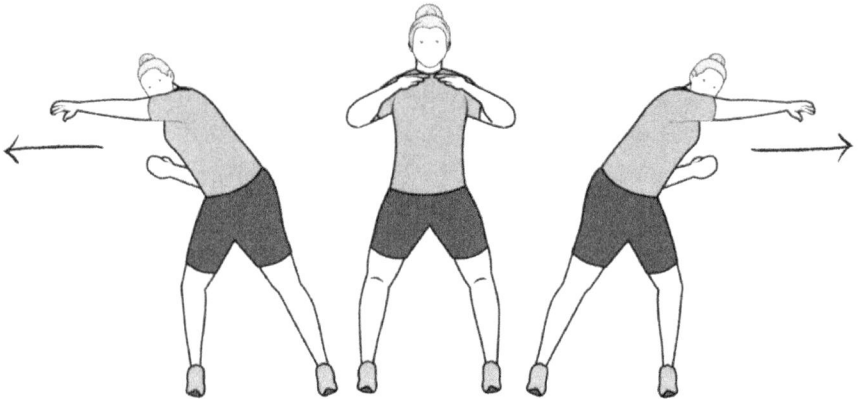

7 STAR SQUAT TO REACH HIGH

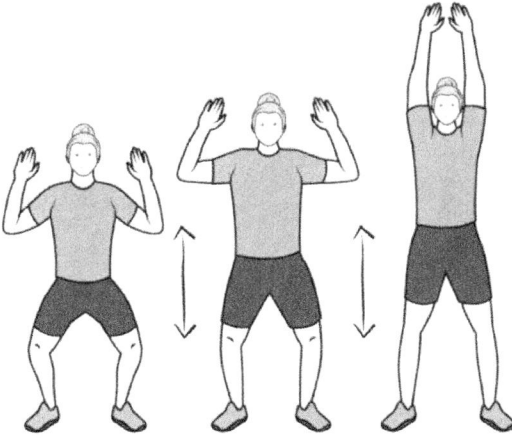

X10
- squat down with hands up as shown

- then squat up + reach hands up

8 ARM CIRCLES

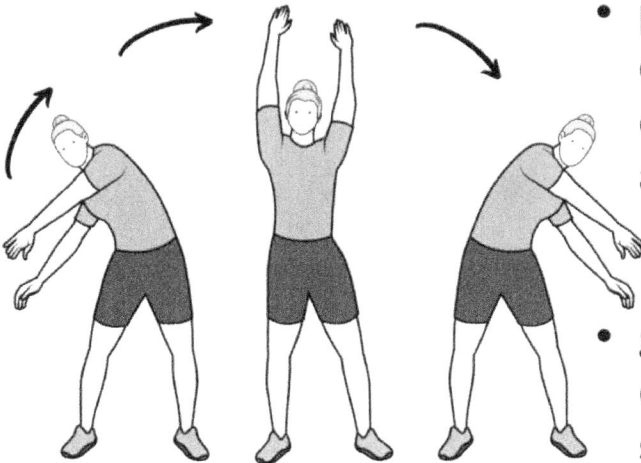

X10 each side
- push hands out + exaggerate arm circles

- go in both directions slowly

9 ROCK TO TALL REACH

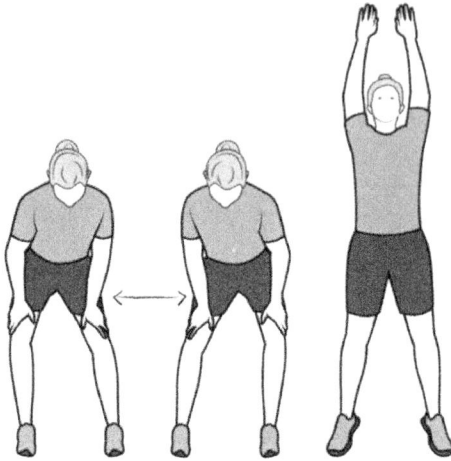

X10

- bend over + rock side to side with hands on legs

- then reach hands tall + reach back

10 UPPERBODY FREESTYLE-SWAY/LOOSEN

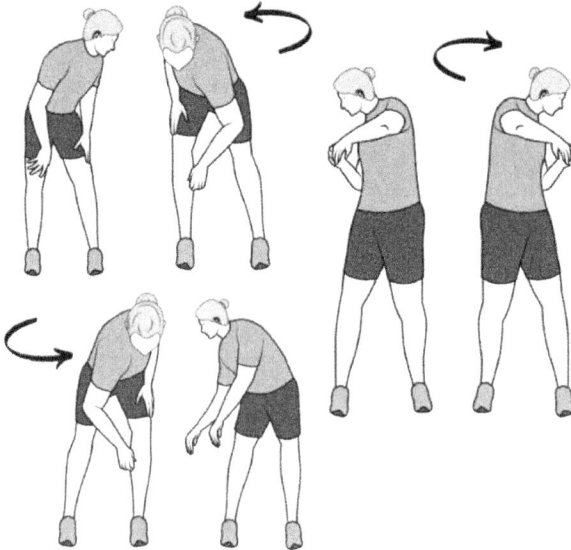

20+ seconds

- freestyle upper-body movements

- (see video demo)

2.3 – WED – BACK RELEASE SUMMARY

1 SHOULDER BLADE ELBOW ROTATIONS

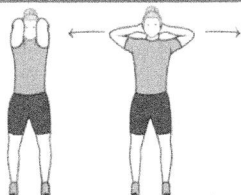

X10

2 HANDS BEHIND HEAD-SIDE TO SIDE

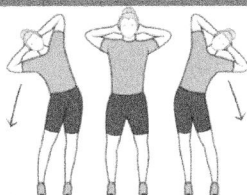

X5 ES

3 CAT/CAMEL STANDING

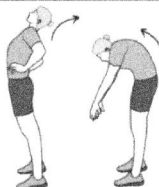

X10

4 OBLIQUE TWIST AND HOLD

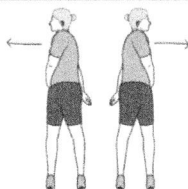

X5 ES

5 TALL TO BEND OVER

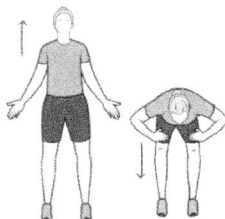

X10

6 SWIMMER REACHES

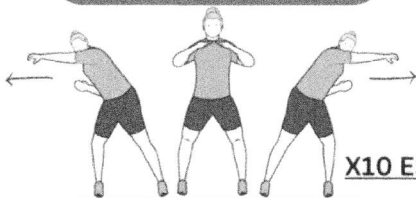

X10 ES

7 STAR SQUAT TO REACH HIGH

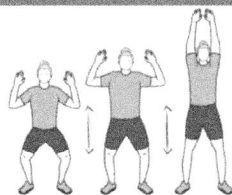

X10

8 ARM CIRCLES

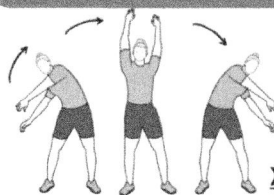

X10 ES

9 ROCK TO TALL REACH

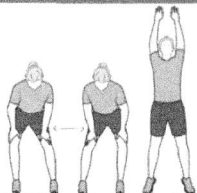

X10

10 UPPER BODY FREESTYLE SWAY/LOOSEN

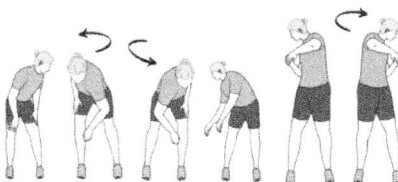

20+ SEC

BRIAN HARDY

2.4 - THURSDAY - CORE STRENGTH

2.4 – THURSDAY – CORE STRENGTH

Welcome to today's **Core Strengthening** workout! Be sure to drink water and warm up correctly before starting. With any core workout, it is **vital** you concentrate on **engaging your core** muscles and keeping a **straight back** and **good posture.** This workout will contain the following:

- A variety of **Abdominal** (core) exercises
- Numerous exercises **lying on your back** or **on all fours**
- **Slow and controlled** movements.
- And more…

There are 10 varying exercises, so it should take approximately 10 minutes to complete. If you can feel your core working and burning, you are doing the exercise correctly. If not, then you could be compensating with other parts of your body. So make sure to always engage your core muscles. If you are doing this workout for the first time, go slowly into each movement, and don't go too far outside your comfort zone.

It is advised to use the **Free Audiobook** (once released) as a guide for these workouts, as it is timed and guides you through each exercise.

Please check the video demonstrations using the **QR code on page 29** for the correct form and technique of each exercise.

Have a good workout!

1 **SINGLE KNEE CRUNCH**

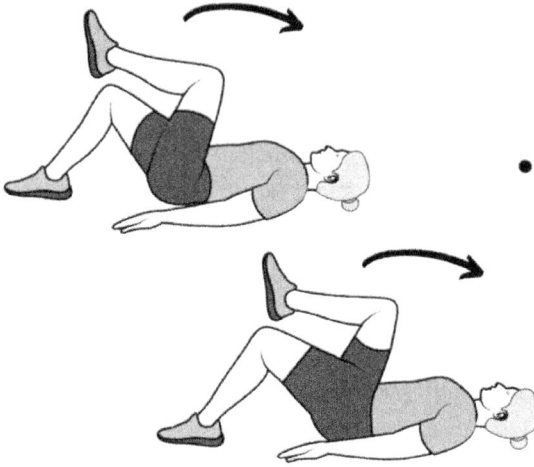

X14 each side

- lie down - arms by side - bend one knee to chest using core

2 **DOUBLE KNEE CRUNCH**

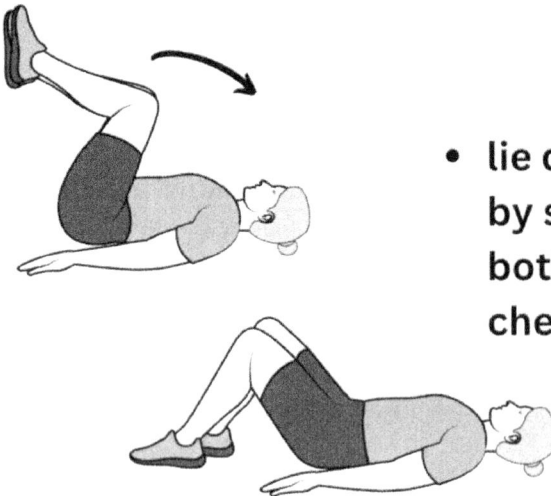

X14

- lie down - arms by side - bend both knees to chest using core

3

KNEE DROPS

X6 each side

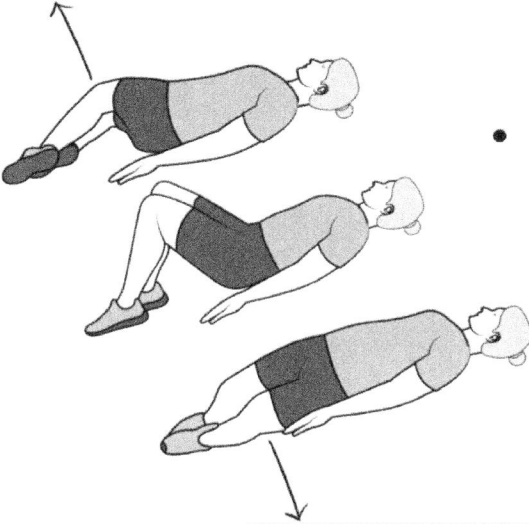

- touch knees + drop them to each side 5 times

4

HEAD CRUNCH UP

X14

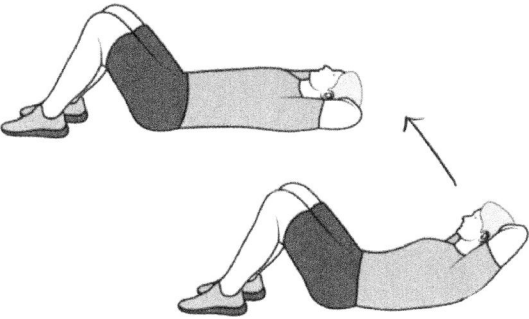

- hands behind head, using core, crunch up

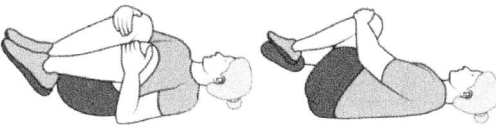

- (Knee hugs + rock for relief after)

5 **FULL SINGLE KNEE CRUNCH**

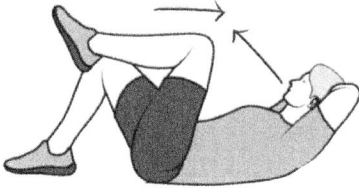

X14 each side

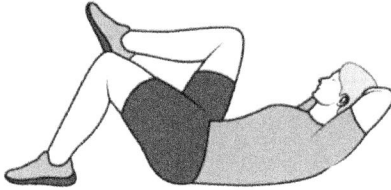

- hands behind head - crunch up with head + crunch one knee to chest

- alternate legs

6 **FULL DOUBLE KNEE CURNCH**

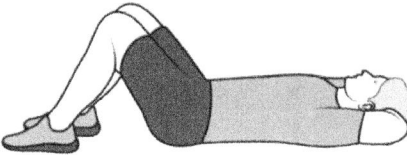

X14

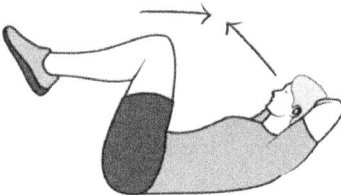

- hands behind head - crunch up with head + crunch both knees to chest

7

HALF DEAD BUG

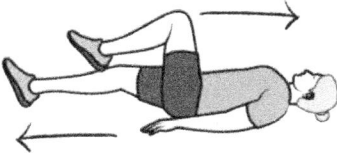

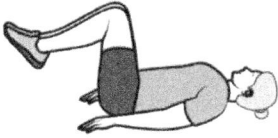

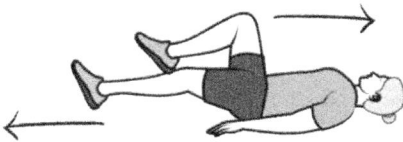

X14 each side

- hands by side - extend one leg out straight + bend other knee up 90 degrees

- change to opposite legs

8

FULL DEAD BUG

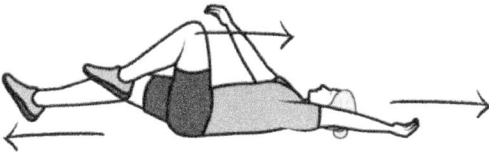

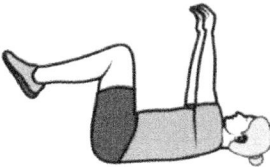

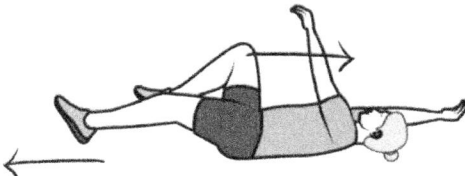

X14

- add in arms - raise arm of bent knee + alternate each side

- (straight leg + opposite straight arm

9 BIRD DOG

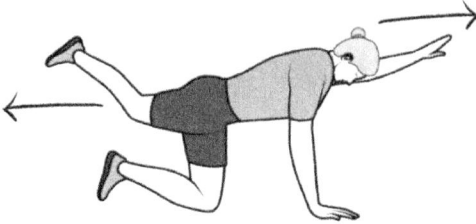

<u>X14 each side</u>
- on all fours - straight left hand out + straight right leg out

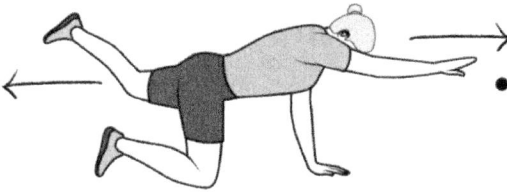

- change + alternate each leg and hand

10 CAT/CAMEL TO CHILDS POSE

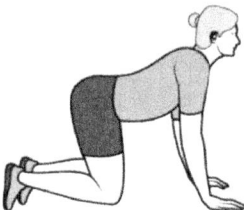

<u>X5</u>
- do the cat + camel pose slowly - then sit into childs pose pushing bum back + arms out in front

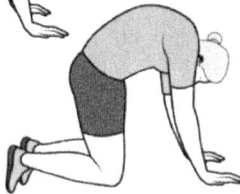

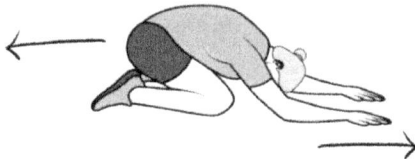

2.4 – THURSDAY – CORE STRENGTH SUMMARY

1 SINGLE KNEE CRUNCH

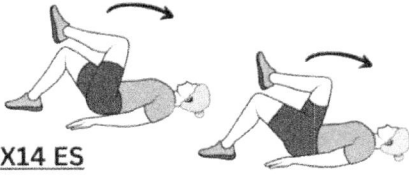

X14 ES

2 DOUBLE KNEE CRUNCH

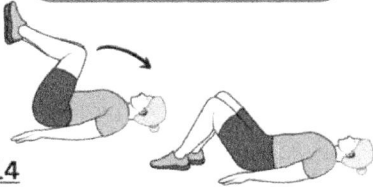

X14

3 KNEE DROPS

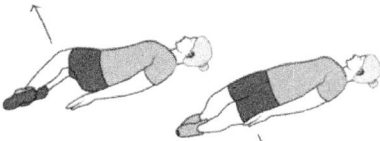

X6 ES

4 HEAD CRUNCH UP (KNEE ROCKS)

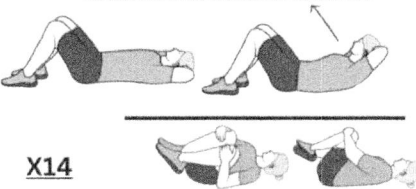

X14

5 FULL SINGLE KNEE CRUNCH

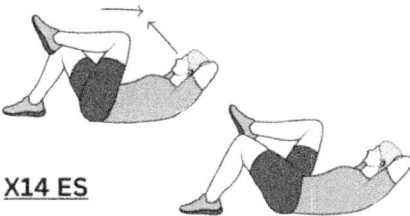

X14 ES

6 FULL DOUBLE KNEE CRUNCH

X14

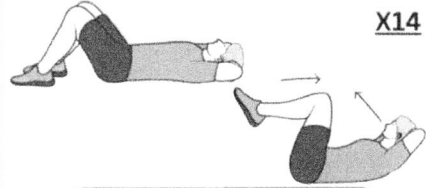

7 HALF DEAD BUG

X14 ES

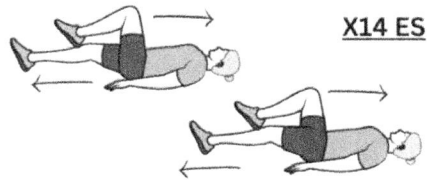

8 FULL DEAD BUG

X14

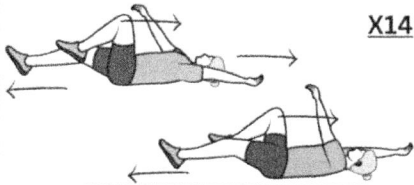

9 BIRD DOG

X14 ES

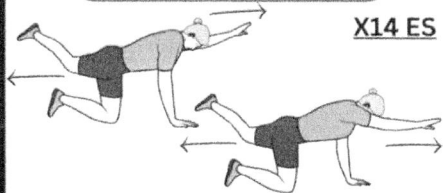

10 CAT/CAMEL TO CHILDS POSE

X5

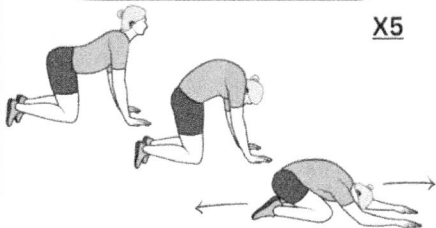

2.5 - FRIDAY - LOWER BODY STRENGTH

2.5 – FRIDAY – LOWER BODY

Welcome to today's **Lower Body Strength** workout! Be sure to drink plenty of water and warm up correctly before starting. Strengthening the leg muscles is vital as you age. Once you begin strengthening these muscles, you may be able to move around with greater ease – improving your overall quality of life! This workout contains several lower-body exercises, such as:

- **Hamstring, groin,** and **quad** muscle exercises
- **Glute, calf,** and **shin** muscle exercises
- **Balance** and **stability** exercises

There are 10 varying exercises with a number of reps to complete for each exercise, so it should take a total of 10 minutes to complete. You can use any chair/table and a small stand or the first step of the stairs for these exercises.

It is advised to use the **Free Audiobook** (once released) as a guide for these workouts, as it is timed and guides you through each exercise.

Please check the video demonstrations using the **QR code on page 29** for correct form and technique. You should never be in pain doing any exercises. Please ensure correct form by stabilizing your core muscles and keeping a bend on your knees and a straight back.

Have a good workout!

1 HAMSTRING KICKS

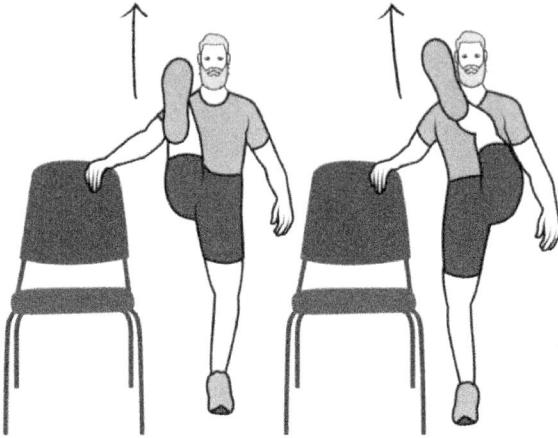

X14 each side

- swinging high kicks
- (hold or wall for balance)

2 STEP UPS

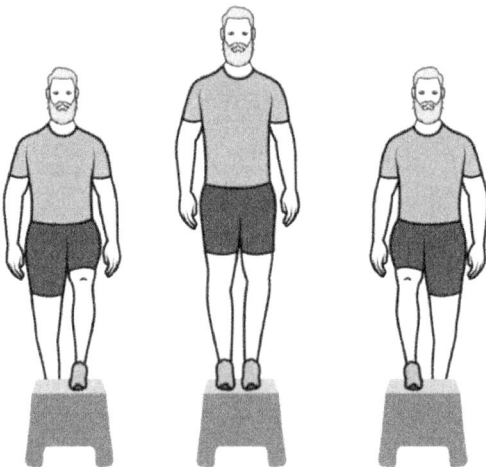

X14 each side

- step ups
- change stepping leg after 14

3 LUNGES

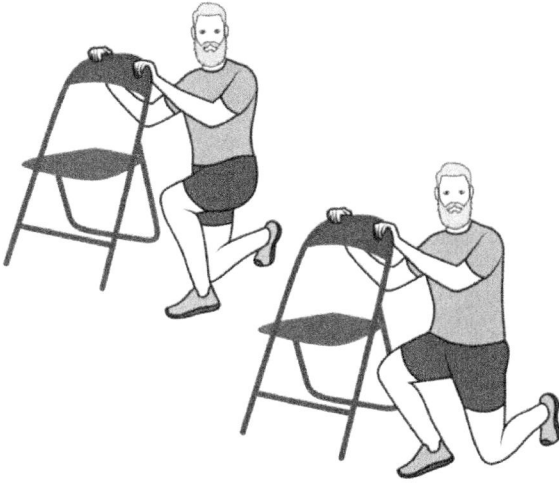

X14 each side

- (use chair or wall for balance)

- Lunge with knee close to or touching ground

4 CALF RAISES (DOUBLE OR SINGLE)

X14 each side

- raise heel(s) off floor + hold for 2 seconds, then drop - (double or single)

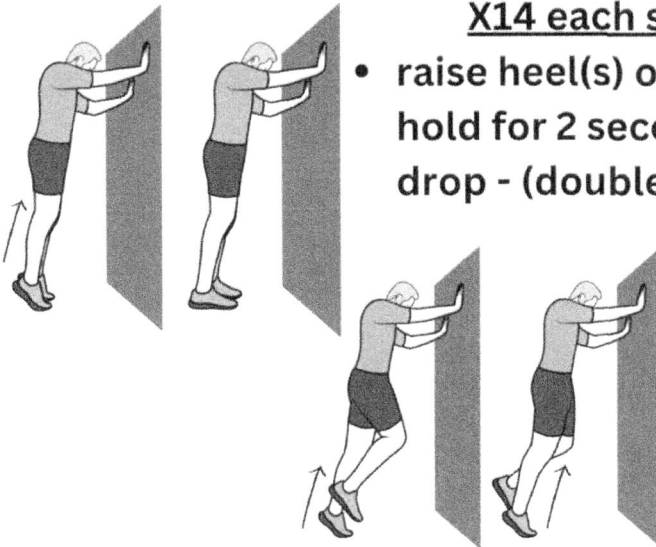

5 SQUATS TO CHAIR

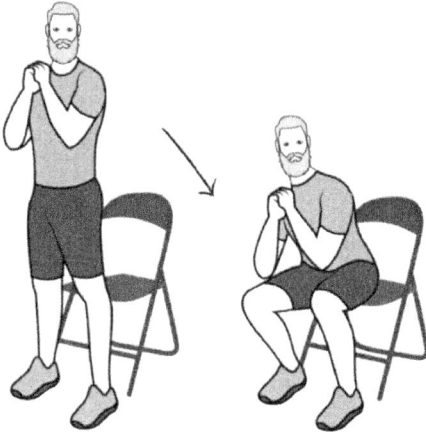

X14

- deep squat to chair
- stand back up

6 BULGARIAN SPLIT SQUAT

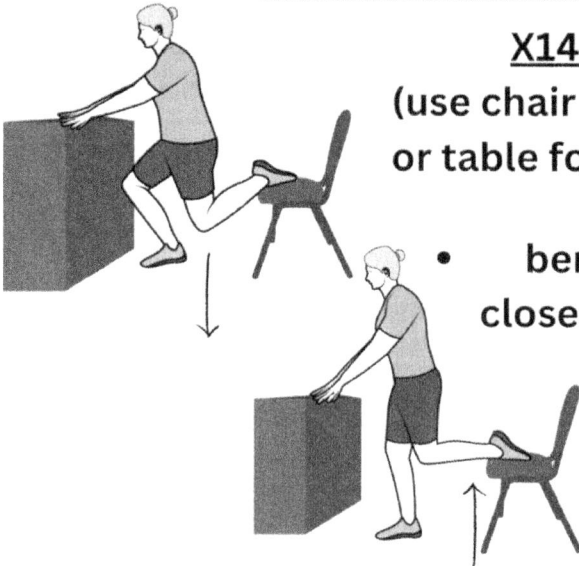

X14 each side
(use chair for foot + wall or table for balance)

- bend knee down close to ground then back up

7 HAMSTRING CURLS

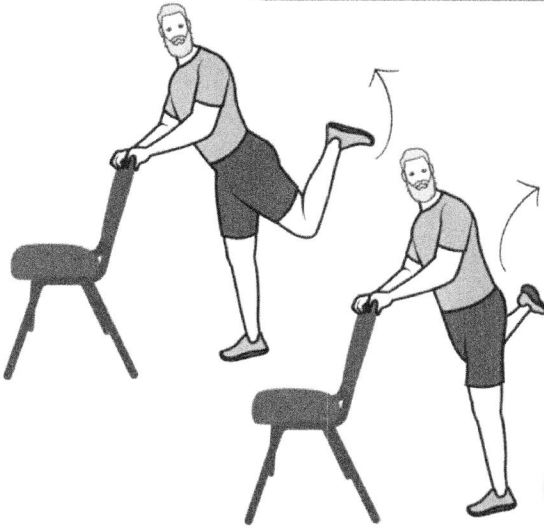

X14 each side
- use chair/wall for balance
- kick back and curl hamstrings left and right

(see video demo)

8 TOE RAISES

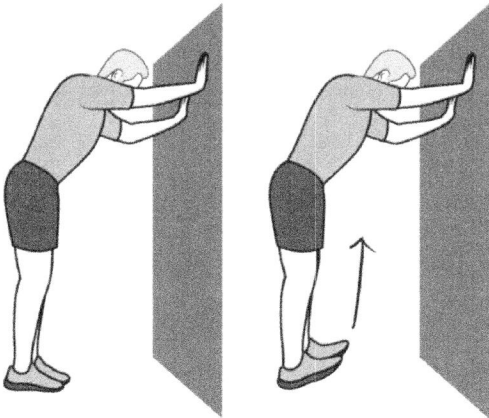

X14

- use wall for balance - point toes to sky and hold for 3 seconds

- (works shin muscles)

9 SIDE LEG RAISES

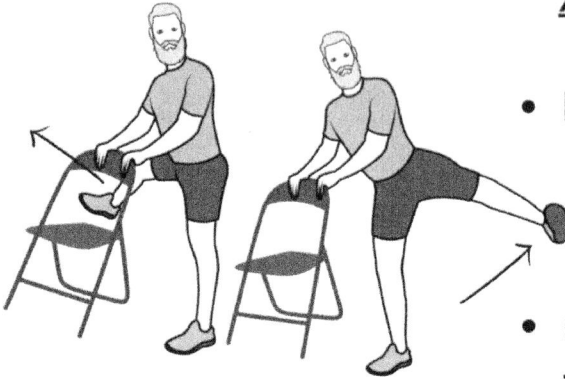

X14 each side

- hold chair/table

- raise foot out to the side and back down

10 GLUTE BRIDGES (DOUBLE OR SINGLE)

DOUBLE

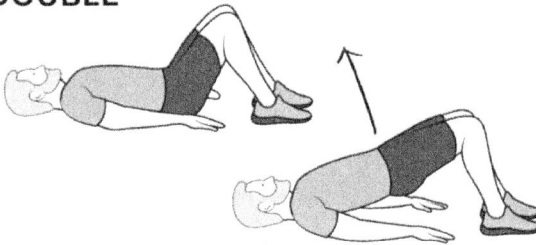

X14

- lie on floor - raise hips to sky + hold for 3 seconds

SINGLE

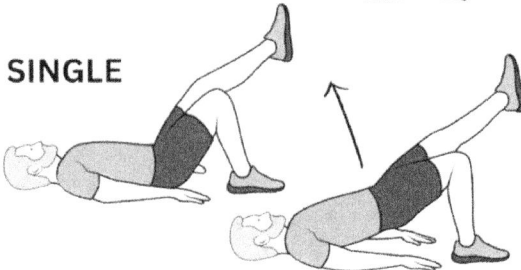

- raise one foot for more difficulty + do each side

2.5 – FRIDAY – LOWER BODY SUMMARY

1 HAMSTRING KICKS

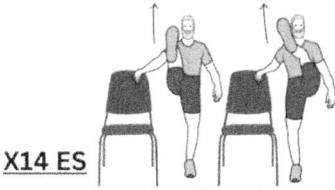

X14 ES

2 STEP-UPS

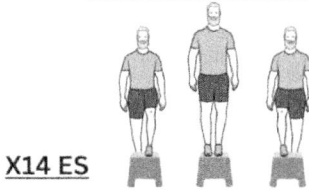

X14 ES

3 LUNGES

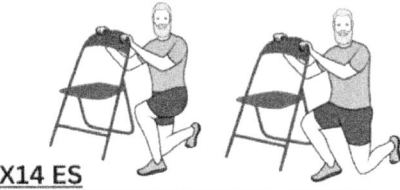

X14 ES

4 CALF RAISES (DOUBLE OR SINGLE)

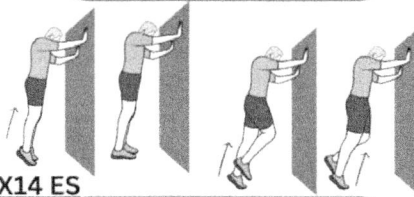

X14 ES

5 SQUATS TO CHAIR

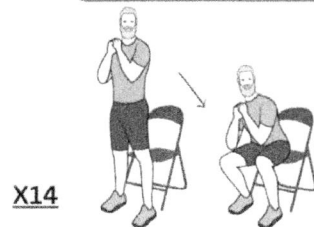

X14

6 BULGARIAN SPLIT SQUAT

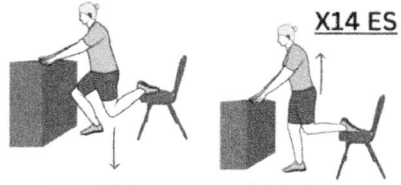

X14 ES

7 HAMSTRING CURLS

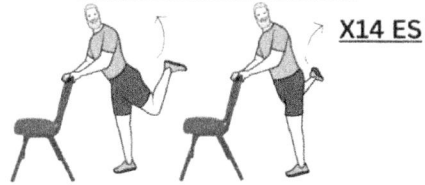

X14 ES

8 TOE RAISES

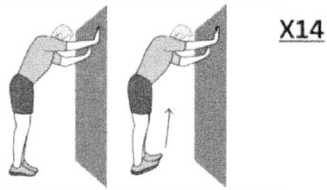

X14

9 SIDE LEG RAISES

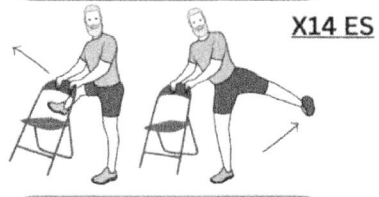

X14 ES

10 GLUTE BRIDGES (DOUBLE OR SINGLE)

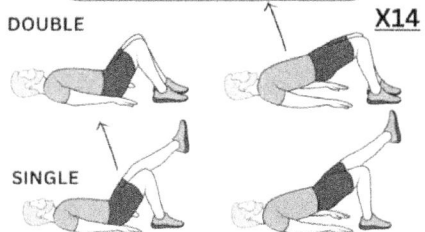

DOUBLE

X14

SINGLE

2.6 - SATURDAY - BOXING CARDIO HIIT 2

2.6 – SATURDAY – BOXING HIIT 2

Welcome to today's **Boxing Cardio HIIT** session! Today is a fun workout, with every workout inspired by boxing training. It's time to unleash your inner **Rocky**! Today's HIIT workout will include:

- **35 seconds** of high-intensity work
- Followed by **25 seconds** of rest before beginning the next exercise/round.
- **Skipping**, **jogging,** and **head movements** to slip and dodge punches
- Different **punch combinations** to deliver the knockout blow to your enemy!

There are 10 varying exercises (or rounds), so it should take a total of 10 minutes to complete. It is advised to use the **Free Audiobook** (once released) as a guide for these workouts, as it is timed and will tell you when 30 seconds are up for each round.

If you are doing this workout for the first time, it is ok to go at a **medium intensity** for the first few rounds. Slowly over time, you can increase the intensity. You want to push yourself just outside your comfort zone each round. Each week you will notice an improvement.

Please check the video demonstrations using the **QR code on page 29** for the correct form and technique of each exercise.

Have a good workout!

1 RUNING ON THE SPOT

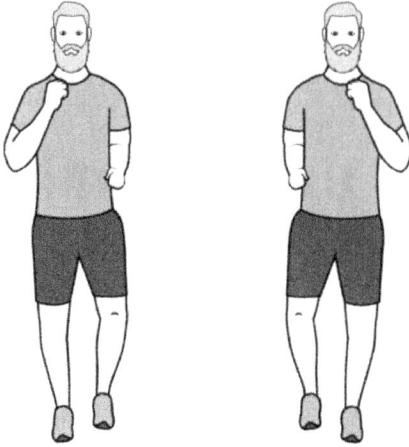

35s on/25s off

- running on the spot

2 JUMPING JACKS

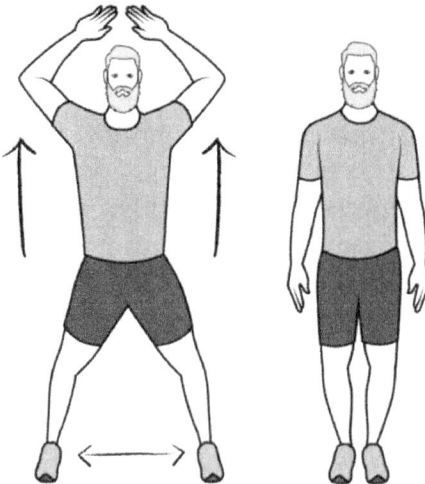

35s on/25s off

- jumping jacks continuously

3   **SKIPPING**

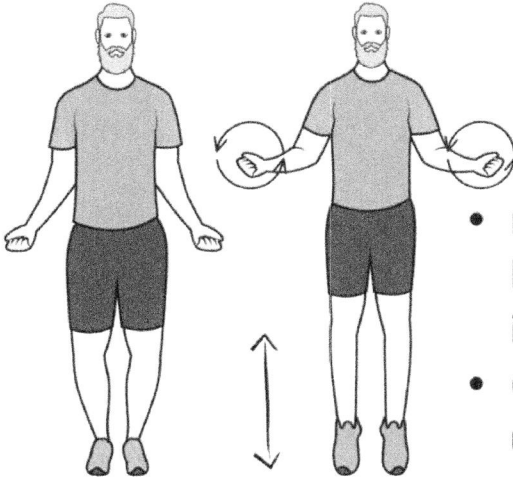

35s on/25s off

- replicate skipping by jumping over an imaginary rope
- (twist wrists + jump up and down)

4   **CROSS PUNCHES**

35s on/25s off

- left hand cross punch + left foot step out
- change to right hand/right foot - repeat

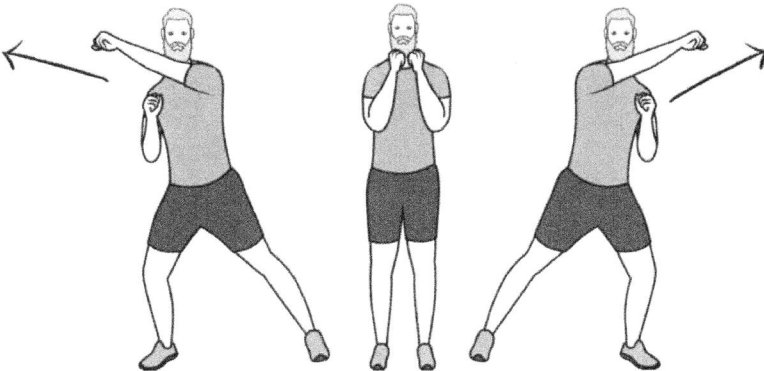

5 SIDE STEP HOOK

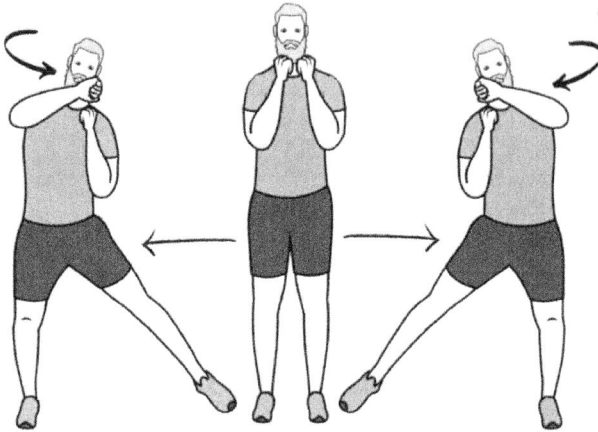

35s on/25s off

- step right - hook right hand - change step left hook left hand

(see video demo)

6 TRICEP FLYS

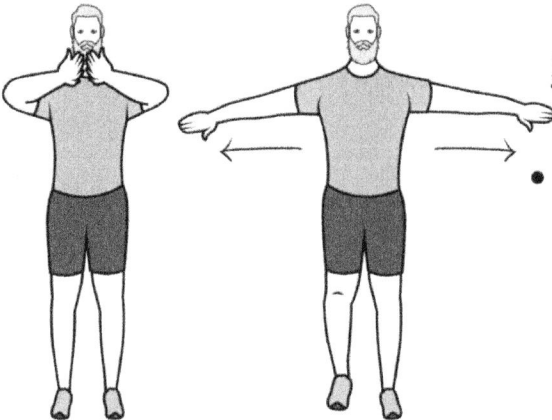

35s on/25s off

- press arms out straight to sides with triceps continuously

7 **DUCK AND WEAVE**

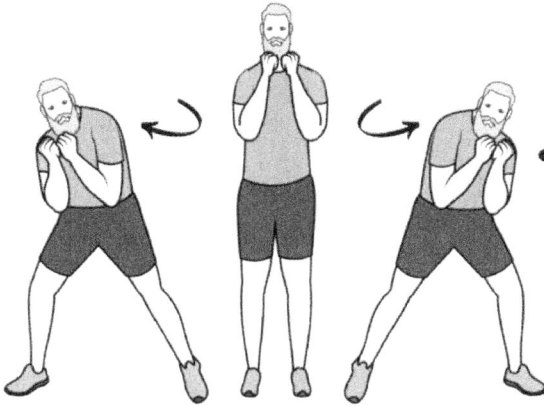

35s on/25s off

- boxers stance - duck right and left with hands up protecting

(see video demo)

8 **UPPERCUTS**

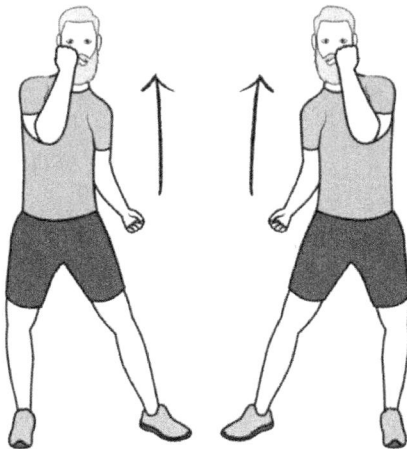

35s on/25s off

- continuous uppercuts right + left

(see video demo)

9 **4 PUNCH COMBO - JAB-JAB-HOOK-HOOK**

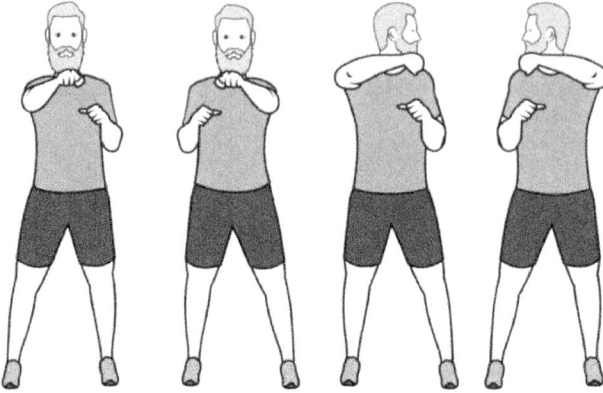

- right jab/
- left jab/
- right hook/
- left hook

repeat

35s on/25s off

10 **RUNNING ON THE SPOT**

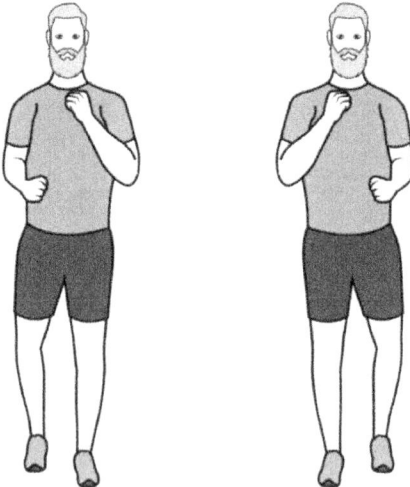

35s on/25s off

- running on the spot
- finish with a fast pace

2.6 – SATURDAY – BOXING HIIT 2 - SUMMARY

1 RUNNING ON THE SPOT

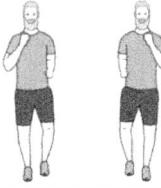

6 TRICEP FLYS

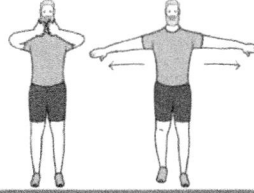

35 SEC WORK | **25 SEC REST**

2 JUMPING JACKS

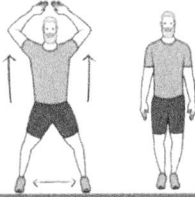

7 DUCK AND WEAVE

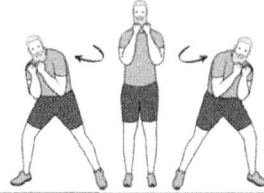

3 SKIPPING

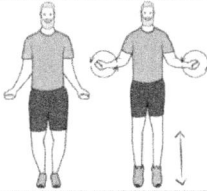

8 UPPERCUTS

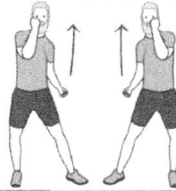

4 CROSS PUNCHES

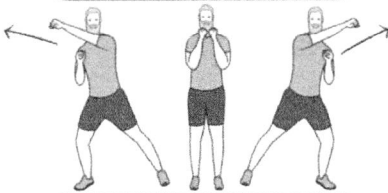

9 4 PUNCH COMBO JAB-JAB-HOOK-HOOK

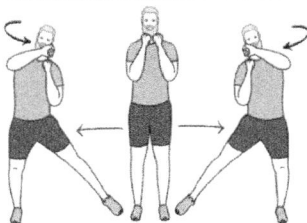

5 SIDE STEP- HOOK

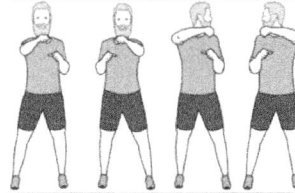

10 RUNNING ON THE SPOT

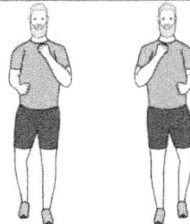

BRIAN HARDY

2.7 - SUNDAY - YOGA

2.7 – SUNDAY – YOGA

Welcome to today's **Yoga** session! Sunday is a day to relax and rejuvenate the mind and body, and this yoga session will help you to do just that. Be sure to drink water and warm up correctly before starting. Yoga is an amazing way to control your breathing, ease your mind, and help the body become used to moving into different positions. Today's yoga session will consist of the following:

- **Slow and controlled** stretches and movements
- **Engaging your core** muscles
- **Controlled breathing** with slow **inhales and exhales**
- **Loosening of the hips, spine,** and much more

There are 10 varying yoga poses, so it should take approximately 10 minutes to complete. This workout is all about calming the mind and body. Follow the steps provided. Some exercises will contain timed holds, while others will have repetitions.

It is advised to use the **Free Audiobook** (once released) as a guide for these workouts, as it is timed and guides you through each exercise.

Please check the video demonstrations using the **QR code on page 29**, for correct form and technique.

Namaste!

1 SIDE REACHES

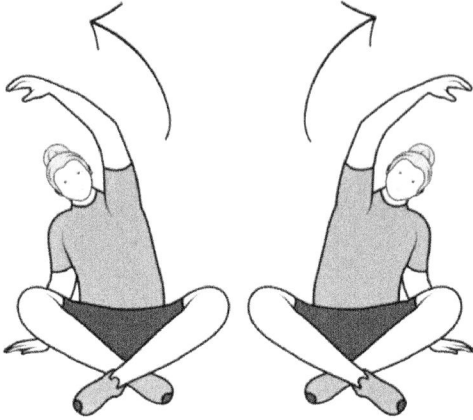

X2 each side

- use other hand for balance - reach over head + hold for 5 seconds each time

2 NECK STRETCHES

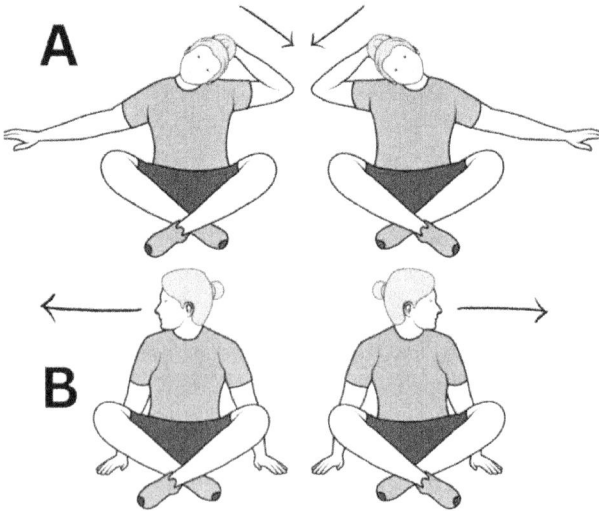

A

B

X2 each side

<u>A</u> - tilt head + light pull down + hold for 5 seconds

<u>B</u> - look to the side + hold for 5 seconds

3 CAT/CAMEL

X5 each
- slow + controlled cat camel poses for 5-10 seconds time

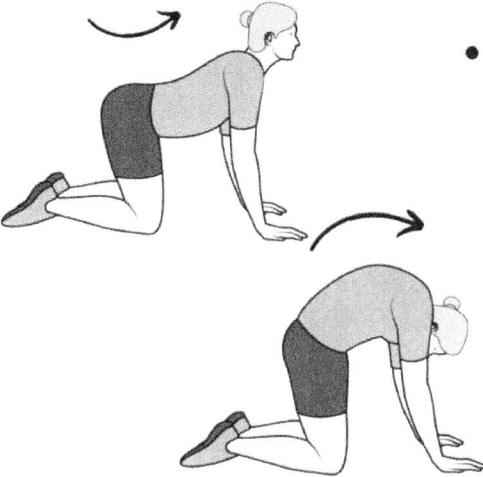

4 CHILDS POSE

30+ seconds
- reach hands forward + sit back into childs pose for 30+ seconds

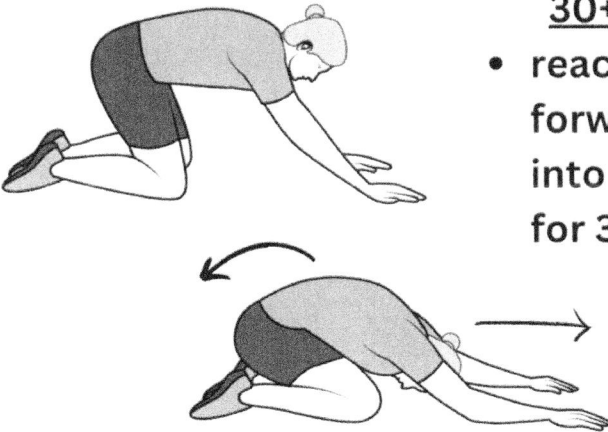

5 — TOE REACH LOOSEN

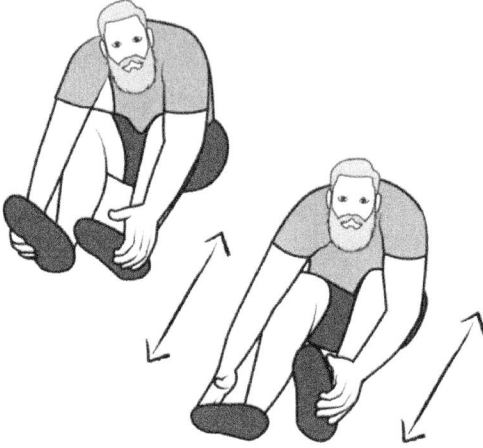

30+ seconds

- bend knees and grab feet - walk out feet for 30+ seconds

6 — HALF LORD TWIST

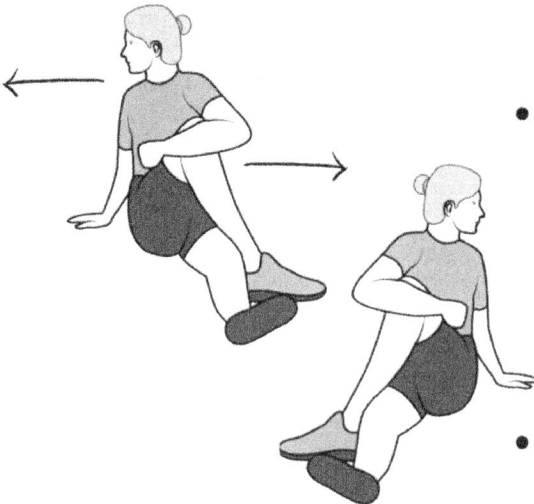

X2 each side

- right leg over left - twist body right as far as possible + hold for 30 seconds

- change to opposite side

7

KNEE HUG AND ROCK

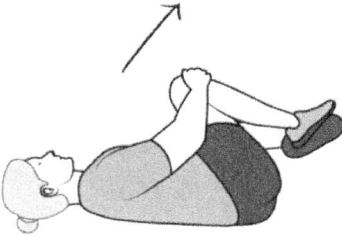

30 seconds

- lie back - hug knees to chest + rock side to side for 30+ seconds

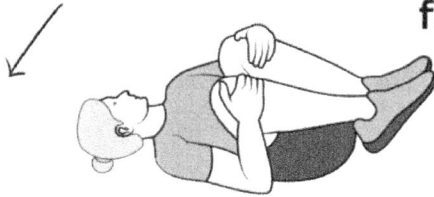

8

GLUTE BRIDGE

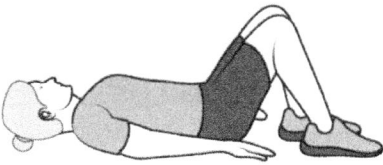

30 seconds

- raise hips to sky for glute bridge + hold for 20-30 seconds

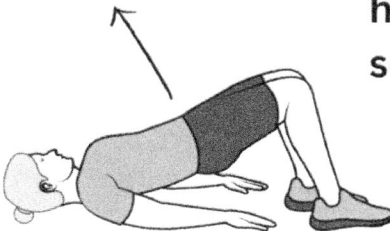

9   HAPPY BABY

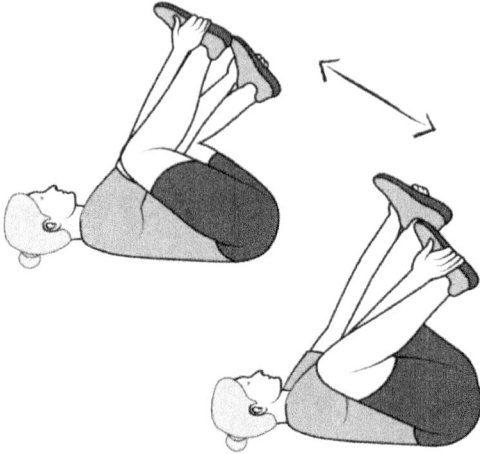

30+ seconds
- bend knees, grab feet + walk out and rock for 30-50 seconds

10   FULL BODY STRETCH

30+ seconds
- lie down flat then stretch arms + legs out for 20 - 30 seconds

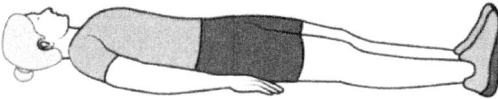

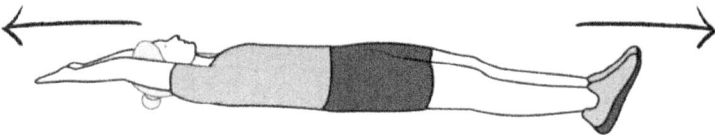

Namaste!

2.7 – SUNDAY – YOGA SUMMARY

1 SIDE REACHES

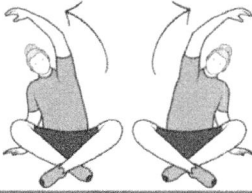

X2 ES
5 SEC

2 NECK STRETCHES

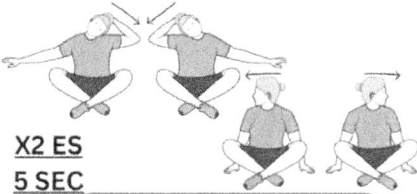

X2 ES
5 SEC

3 CAT/CAMEL

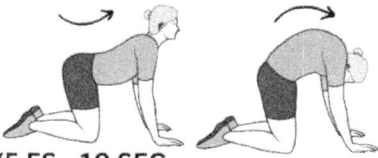

X5 ES - 10 SEC

4 CHILDS POSE

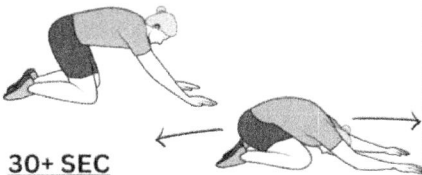

30+ SEC

5 TOE REACH LOOSEN

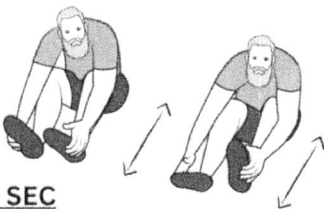

30+ SEC

6 HALF LORD TWIST

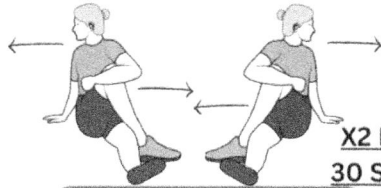

X2 ES
30 SEC

7 KNEE HUG AND ROCK

30+ SEC

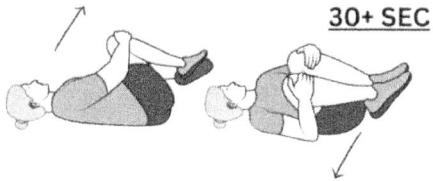

8 GLUTE BRIDGE

30 SEC

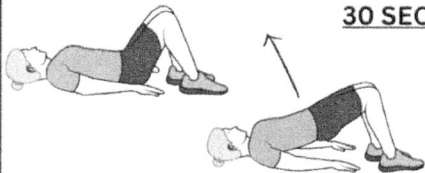

9 HAPPY BABY

30+ SEC

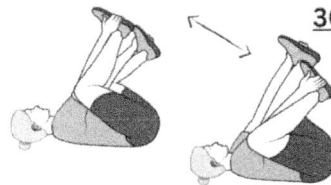

10 FULL BODY STRETCH

30+ SEC

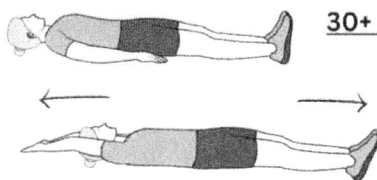

Namaste!

CONCLUSION

And so we come to the end of *'10-Minute Home Workouts for Seniors.* I truly enjoyed every minute of creating this workout book. I was inspired to create a standing workout edition after the amazing positive feedback I received about my *'10-Minute Chair Exercises for Seniors* from people all over the world. I was overwhelmed by the number of positive emails and messages I received. I also tried to make adjustments and improvements based on some recommendations. Overall, I kept it simple and direct as that seems to be what people enjoyed about book one. Thank you all once again from the bottom of my heart. It would mean a lot if you could also leave a brief review for this book (see page 95 for the link). That way, the book can become accessible to others who could benefit from the routines and improve their health. I appreciate you all.

It's extraordinary how much your physical and mental well-being can improve in just a few weeks of sticking to a routine and being consistent.

I hope this book helped you recognize the advantages of maintaining strong muscles and a healthy heart as you grow older. It's so important to stay mobile for as long as possible, so you can enjoy time with your loved ones and play around grandchildren. For your self-esteem, it's also vital not to constantly depend on others to assist you in your daily tasks. Of course, there is nothing wrong with this, and there will come a time in everyone's life when you will need assistance, but you should always aim to delay this day for as long as possible. There really is no age limit to how long you can stay mobile and active. We have all heard stories or know someone active, energetic, and full of life well into their 90s and beyond!

While maintaining physical fitness is essential, a healthy state of mind is equally important. Regular exercise can also lead to significant mental benefits. Concentrating on proper form and technique for each exercise can greatly enhance your mental capacity.

Another thing I highly recommend is looking into yoga classes nearby you. Yoga has amazing benefits for your body and mind, helping you to relax and stay calm while getting stronger and more flexible at the same time. There are tons of fantastic yoga communities out there.

Developing confidence in your body and improving your stability and mobility will allow you to continue completing simple tasks effortlessly. It doesn't matter where you start, even if it's been a year or 10 years since you last exercised! You'll be surprised by how magnificent the human body is at adapting to a new routine and environment. Once the body gets to grip and understands that you are working out for 10 minutes a day, it will simply adapt to this habit after a short while. With slow and steady progression, there is no limit to how far you can improve your mobility and health over a 3- or 6-month period. You may feel like a new person!

My goal has been achieved if I assisted you from doing little to no exercise to even 2 or 3 workouts a week. If you are finding the workouts easy and are advancing quickly, feel free to make your own changes to make the workouts even more challenging.

I created this book and my other *10-Minute Chair Exercises* book for a no-nonsense, simple, and practical workout alternative for senior citizens. I hope the uncomplex nature of the book appealed to you and that you acquired some new insights and knowledge.

At the beginning of this book, I promised that if you stick to these workouts consistently, there's every chance you will have a new spring in your step and experience newfound energy. I truly hope that has been the case for you. Thank you for taking the time to read this book, and I wish you continued health and joy in the years ahead!

BRIAN HARDY

REFERENCES

Bolton, K., Kremer, P., & Jefferis, B. J. (2021). Strength training and older adults: A meta-analysis and meta-regression. Journal of Musculoskeletal and Neuronal Interactions, 21(2), 269-281.

Burgin, T. (n.d.). What is Yoga? https://www.yogabasics.com/learn/yoga-101-an-introduction/what-is-yoga/

Clear, J. (2021). Atomic habits: Tiny changes, remarkable results: An easy & proven way to build Good Habits & Break Bad Ones. CELA.

Get fit while you sit with chair exercises. Brain and Life Magazine - Trusted by Neurologists. (n.d.). Retrieved October 23, 2022, from https://www.brainandlife.org/articles/get-fit-while-you-sit-with-chair-exercises#:~:text=A%202019%20study%20in%20the,significantly%20decreased%20fear%20of%20falling.

Hardy, B. (2022). 10-Minute Chair Exercises for Seniors; 7 Simple Workout Routines for Each Day of the Week. 70+ Illustrated Exercises with Video demos for Cardio, Core, Yoga, Back Stretching, and more. Independent.

Harvard Medical School (March 2022). The importance of stretching. https://www.health.harvard.edu/staying-healthy/the-importance-of-stretching

Harvard Medical School (September 2018). Understanding and improving core strength. Understanding and improving core strength - Harvard Health

Mayo Clinic. (February 2022). Stretching: Focus on flexibility. https://www.mayoclinic.org/healthy-lifestyle/fitness/in-depth/stretching/art-20047931

National Center for Complementary and Integrative Health. (April 2021). Yoga: What You Need to Know. https://www.nccih.nih.gov/health/yoga-what-you-need-to-know

Pinckard, K., Baskin, K., & Stanford, K. (June 2019). Effects of Exercise to Improve Cardiovascular Health. Frontiers in cardiovascular medicine. https://doi.org/10.3389/fcvm.2019.00069

ABOUT AUTHOR

Brian Hardy is a high-school coach with numerous credentials in both his coaching and playing career. Brian has coached successful high school and local soccer and basketball teams for 10+ years. He has also been involved in elite-level sports as an athlete himself, performing at national games in athletics, soccer, and basketball. Brian has been studying Strength and conditioning and sports psychology for several years. He has been involved in developing numerous fitness programs, such as aerobic fitness, speed, mobility programs, and more. He has also been practicing yoga and meditation for years and intends to become a yoga instructor in time. Brian is always seeking to learn from the best and learn the latest knowledge and science in the sports and fitness industry. This is why Brian sought assistance with Michael Sheehan for this book. As mentioned in the book, Michael is a qualified chartered physiotherapist, working with professional athletes and continuously running mobility and workout classes for all age groups. Michael's whole focus is centered around rehabilitation and injury prevention, making him the perfect fit for this book.

Printed in Great Britain
by Amazon